A Build Confidence Book for Women

CRAFTED BY SKRIUWER

Copyright © 2024 by Skriuwer.

All rights reserved. No part of this book may be used or reproduced in any form whatsoever without written permission except in the case of brief quotations in critical articles or reviews.

For more information, contact : **kontakt@skriuwer.com** (www.skriuwer.com)

TABLE OF CONTENTS

CHAPTER 1: UNDERSTANDING CONFIDENCE

- *Defining confidence as self-trust rather than perfection*
- *Recognizing normal insecurities and how to address them*
- *Foundations for healthy self-esteem*

CHAPTER 2: THE INNER CRITIC AND HOW TO OVERCOME IT

- *Identifying negative self-talk and its sources*
- *Techniques for challenging harmful beliefs*
- *Replacing criticism with empowering affirmations*

CHAPTER 3: SELF-AWARENESS AND ACCEPTANCE

- *Recognizing your strengths, flaws, and triggers*
- *Embracing self-compassion and personal honesty*
- *Using reflection to guide healthier choices*

CHAPTER 4: SETTING GOALS AND BUILDING MOTIVATION

- *Turning broad desires into specific, achievable targets*
- *Creating step-by-step action plans*
- *Staying motivated through rewards and accountability*

CHAPTER 5: SELF-CARE FOR MENTAL AND EMOTIONAL HEALTH

- *Balancing rest, exercise, and emotional well-being*
- *Practical daily habits to reduce stress and anxiety*
- *Realigning personal needs with supportive routines*

CHAPTER 6: HEALTHY BOUNDARIES AND ASSERTIVENESS

- Distinguishing supportive relationships from toxic ones
- Speaking up confidently without guilt
- Protecting time and energy through respectful limits

CHAPTER 7: EMOTIONAL RESILIENCE

- Understanding resilience as the ability to bounce back
- Building habits that foster mental and emotional strength
- Turning challenges into opportunities for growth

CHAPTER 8: POWER OF POSITIVE THINKING

- Shifting your mindset to see possibilities over problems
- Using affirmations and gratitude to nurture optimism
- Balancing hopeful outlooks with realistic actions

CHAPTER 9: STRENGTHENING YOUR COMMUNICATION SKILLS

- Practicing active listening and respectful dialogue
- Speaking up effectively in personal and professional settings
- Resolving conflicts calmly while staying true to yourself

CHAPTER 10: MANAGING FEAR AND STRESS

- Understanding common stress triggers and responses
- Simple coping techniques like mindfulness and structured breaks
- Transforming anxiety into constructive problem-solving energy

CHAPTER 11: EMBRACING YOUR UNIQUE QUALITIES

- Celebrating personal traits and cultural backgrounds
- Overcoming the pressure to conform
- Discovering self-acceptance and authentic expression

CHAPTER 12: BUILDING POSITIVE HABITS

- Identifying key habits for lasting confidence
- Breaking down behaviors into daily, doable actions
- Tracking progress and adjusting strategies over time

CHAPTER 13: RELATIONSHIPS AND SOCIAL SUPPORT

- Cultivating healthy friendships, family ties, and community bonds
- Handling conflicts with empathy and open communication
- Understanding the value of nurturing a support network

CHAPTER 14: OVERCOMING COMMON OBSTACLES

- Tackling financial, emotional, and time-related barriers
- Turning failures into lessons that fuel new growth
- Preparing flexible solutions for recurring challenges

CHAPTER 15: THE ROLE OF SPIRITUALITY OR MINDFULNESS

- Finding inner peace and purpose through reflection or faith
- Using meditation and mindful habits to reduce stress
- Strengthening emotional stability with spiritual practices

CHAPTER 16: CAREER AND AMBITION

- Defining your version of professional success
- Navigating biases, negotiating promotions, and continuous learning
- Balancing drive with personal fulfillment and well-being

CHAPTER 17: BALANCING DIFFERENT ROLES IN LIFE

- Juggling responsibilities as a professional, caregiver, friend, and more
- Time management techniques and setting practical boundaries
- Avoiding burnout by prioritizing self-care and realistic goals

CHAPTER 18: MENTORING AND GUIDING OTHERS

- Building supportive, growth-focused relationships
- Methods for effective communication and problem-solving
- Empowering future leaders and sharing knowledge generously

CHAPTER 19: CRAFTING A PERSONAL DEVELOPMENT PLAN

- Defining clear, measurable goals aligned with core values
- Breaking down ambitions into step-by-step actions
- Staying accountable, tracking progress, and refining over time

CHAPTER 20: CELEBRATING PROGRESS AND PLANNING FOR THE FUTURE

- Recognizing and honoring both internal and external achievements
- Creating new goals from completed milestones
- Sustaining confidence through continued growth and hope

CHAPTER 1

Understanding Confidence

1.1 What Is Confidence?

Confidence is a feeling inside you that says, "I can do this." It is the belief that you have the skills, knowledge, or ability to handle life's tasks or challenges. Even if you are unsure how something will turn out, having confidence means you trust yourself to figure things out. You do not need to be perfect to be confident; you only need to believe you can keep trying until you succeed.

Some people think confidence means you must be loud or showy. That is not true. You do not have to brag or stand out in every crowd to be confident. Confidence can be quiet and calm. A confident person can be the one who quietly does her work, helps others, or simply believes she can make it through tough times. Confidence shows up in many ways—through your actions, your voice, and even your body language.

When you believe in yourself, you are more likely to take healthy risks. You might try for a better job, speak your ideas in a meeting, or stand up for a friend. Confidence helps you move forward instead of staying stuck in fear or self-doubt. At its core, confidence is about trusting that you can learn, adapt, and keep going, no matter the situation.

1.2 Why Does Confidence Matter?

Confidence makes life more fulfilling. When you believe in yourself, you can:

1. **Try New Things**: *You are more open to new experiences and less scared of failing. For example, if you have never tried painting before, you will be more likely to give it a shot if you feel confident that you can learn.*
2. **Express Your Thoughts**: *You are more willing to speak up in discussions or share your ideas at work. You do not shy away from offering your opinion because you trust that it might help.*

3. **Enjoy Healthier Relationships**: Confidence allows you to set boundaries and respect other people's boundaries too. You do not feel threatened by others' success, and you can celebrate with them. Confident people often build more positive and supportive relationships.
4. **Handle Criticism Better**: Confident people can take feedback in a healthier way. They do not fall apart when they get negative comments or suggestions. Instead, they see it as a chance to learn.
5. **Lead a Happier Life**: When you trust yourself, you experience less stress. You also feel more in control, which can lead to a more satisfying and calm life.

1.3 The Difference Between Confidence and Arrogance

Sometimes people mix up confidence with arrogance. They might think that someone who is sure of herself is also stuck-up or full of herself. However, there is a clear difference:

- **Arrogance**: This is when a person believes she is better than everyone else. She might brag excessively or look down on others. Arrogant people often blame others for mistakes and rarely admit their own shortcomings.
- **Confidence**: This is when you believe in your ability to grow, learn, and achieve goals without looking down on others. A confident person knows she is not perfect, but she is also aware she can improve over time. She respects other people's talents and skills.

Having confidence does not mean you never make mistakes. In fact, admitting your mistakes and being willing to learn from them is a strong sign of healthy confidence.

1.4 How Self-Esteem Ties Into Confidence

Self-esteem is how you see yourself overall—your sense of self-worth. It is like the foundation of a building. If your self-esteem is strong, it supports your confidence. If it is weak, you might find it harder to believe in yourself, even when you have talents or skills. Here is how they connect:

- **Self-Esteem**: Believing you are valuable and worthy of good things in life. You accept yourself, flaws and all.

- **Confidence**: Trusting your abilities or knowledge in specific tasks or situations.

You can have decent self-esteem but still lack confidence in certain skills, or vice versa. For example, you may deeply respect yourself as a person (strong self-esteem) yet feel nervous about public speaking (lower confidence in that area). Over time, improving your self-esteem in a broad sense can help your confidence grow in many areas.

1.5 Factors That Shape Your Confidence

Confidence is not something you are born with. It often develops over time due to many factors:

1. **Early Experiences**: How your parents or caregivers spoke to you when you were a child can impact your confidence level. If they encouraged you and praised your efforts, you may have grown up feeling more capable. If they were overly critical, you might doubt yourself more as an adult.
2. **Environment**: The people you surround yourself with can either lift you up or bring you down. Positive, supportive friends often help build your confidence, while toxic, negative influences can lower it.
3. **Achievements**: Success in different areas of life helps build your confidence. This might mean getting a good grade, performing well in a sports event, or learning a new skill. Each win shows you what you are capable of.
4. **Failures**: Oddly enough, failing at something can also improve your confidence, if you approach it with a learning mindset. When you fail, you learn what does not work. Then you can make changes and do better next time. Seeing yourself bounce back from setbacks can be a big confidence booster.
5. **Personal Traits**: Some people are naturally more outgoing, while others are shy. This can affect how they show confidence. However, both extroverts and introverts can be confident. It is simply about learning to believe in yourself, regardless of your personality.

1.6 Common Myths About Confidence

- **Myth #1: You Have to Be Born With It**
  Reality: Confidence is a skill you can learn. Yes, some people have an easier time feeling confident, but anyone can build it through practice.
- **Myth #2: Confident People Never Fail**
  Reality: Everyone fails at some point. Confident people do not let failure define them. They see failure as an opportunity to improve.
- **Myth #3: Confidence Means You Never Feel Scared**
  Reality: Even the most confident individuals feel fear. The difference is they do not let fear stop them from trying. They move forward in spite of the fear.
- **Myth #4: You Must Always Be the Center of Attention**
  Reality: Many confident people are quiet. They do not need the spotlight to feel good about themselves. They know their worth, whether they are in front of a crowd or not.

1.7 Benefits of Building Your Confidence

Feeling more confident has many positive effects on your life. Here are a few you may notice:

1. **Better Decision-Making**: When you trust yourself, you are less likely to second-guess every choice. You can weigh your options and choose a path without endless worry.
2. **Increased Resilience**: Confidence helps you bounce back from failure or disappointment. You know that a single setback does not mean you are incapable.
3. **Improved Mental Health**: Constant self-doubt can lead to anxiety or depression. Confidence brings more balance, reducing stress over time.
4. **Greater Happiness**: Believing in yourself leads to a sense of accomplishment. This can improve your overall mood and make you happier day by day.
5. **More Opportunities**: Employers, friends, and even community groups tend to trust people who trust themselves. This can open doors to jobs, partnerships, and social activities that might not have been available otherwise.

1.8 Small Daily Steps to Boost Confidence

A few daily habits can help you slowly build a more confident mindset:

1. **Positive Self-Talk**: Start your day by telling yourself, "I am capable and strong." Simple statements like this can set a positive tone for the rest of your day.
2. **Set Achievable Goals**: Give yourself small tasks you can finish. Each success, no matter how minor, proves you can get things done.
3. **Celebrate Wins**: Did you complete a workout? Did you speak up in class or a meeting? Celebrate it! Recognize your progress and let yourself feel proud.
4. **Learn Continuously**: Try reading a new book, watching a tutorial, or practicing a skill every day. Learning helps you see your growth and builds trust in your abilities.
5. **Reflect on Your Day**: Before bedtime, think about what went well. Write it in a journal or just talk it out with yourself. This helps you focus on positives rather than negatives.

1.9 Practical Example: Sarah's Story

Sarah used to be afraid of speaking up at her job. She worried that her coworkers would judge her ideas. Over time, she practiced speaking in small, low-pressure situations, like team huddles. She also prepared ahead of time by writing down a few talking points. After a few weeks, she noticed she was not shaking as much before she spoke. Her heart still pounded, but her words came out more smoothly. Because of her effort, Sarah's manager asked her to help lead a project, giving her a chance to show even more of her abilities. Sarah learned that taking small steps can open bigger opportunities, which in turn boosted her confidence.

1.10 The Role of Self-Reflection

A big part of growing your confidence is getting to know yourself well. This includes noticing your strengths, weaknesses, and triggers. You can do this by:

1. **Journaling**: Write about your day, your feelings, and your dreams. This helps you see patterns in your thoughts and actions.

2. **Asking for Feedback**: Talk to people you trust—friends, family, or mentors. Ask them what they see as your strengths and areas for improvement. Their answers can guide you to a better self-understanding.
3. **Meditation or Quiet Time**: Spend a few minutes each day sitting quietly, focusing on your breath, and letting thoughts pass by without judgment. It might feel awkward at first, but it can help you become more aware of what is happening inside your mind.

1.11 Building a Foundation for Future Growth

Think of confidence as a house you are building. Your thoughts and beliefs about yourself form the foundation. If you start with a strong base—that is, healthy self-esteem and positive self-talk—then the rest of the structure stands sturdier against harsh weather. In future chapters, we will discuss how to handle self-criticism, set goals, and practice self-care. All these elements work together like bricks and beams, helping you create a supportive home inside yourself.

1.12 Exercises to Try

1. **Mirror Talk**: Stand in front of a mirror, look yourself in the eyes, and say something kind. It might feel silly at first, but it can slowly train your brain to see yourself in a more positive light.
2. **Confidence Journal**: Each day, write down one thing you did that required some level of courage, even if it was small. Over time, you will have a list of achievements to remind you of your progress.
3. **Skill Building**: Pick one skill you want to improve—cooking, writing, running, anything. Spend 15 minutes a day working on it. Watch how regular practice boosts your confidence in that area.
4. **Small Acts of Bravery**: Do something that feels slightly outside your comfort zone, like introducing yourself to a neighbor or offering a new idea at work. Each small step teaches you that you are capable of more than you might think.

CHAPTER 2

The Inner Critic and How to Overcome It

2.1 Meeting Your Inner Critic

Almost everyone has an inner critic. This is the voice in your head that points out your mistakes, doubts your abilities, and sometimes calls you names. It might say, "You are not smart enough," or "You will fail again, so why try?" The inner critic often tries to protect you from disappointment by keeping you from taking risks. But in doing so, it also holds you back.

It is important to recognize that this voice is just one part of your thoughts. It may feel powerful, but it is not the final judge of your worth or capabilities. Realizing that you can question this voice is the first step to managing it.

2.2 Why We Have an Inner Critic

The inner critic can develop for many reasons:

1. **Past Criticism**: *If you grew up hearing negative messages—like you were too lazy or not talented—these words might have stuck in your head. Over time, you learned to believe them and repeat them to yourself.*
2. **Fear of Failure**: *Sometimes we criticize ourselves because we do not want to fail. The critic thinks that by pointing out possible mistakes, it can help us avoid them. But too often, it just stops us from even trying.*
3. **Comparison With Others**: *When you see others doing well, you might feel inferior. Your inner critic jumps in to say, "See, you are not as good as them." This leads you to judge yourself harshly.*
4. **Perfectionism**: *If you have high standards for yourself, you might never feel satisfied with your work. The inner critic gets louder each time you fall short of your ideal perfection.*

2.3 Signs Your Inner Critic Is Taking Over

How do you know when your inner critic is running the show? Here are some signs:

- You talk down to yourself in your mind. You use harsh words you would never say to a friend.
- You avoid trying new things because you are sure you will fail.
- You think about your past mistakes again and again, feeling guilty or ashamed.
- You find it hard to accept compliments, often brushing them off or thinking people are just being polite.

If you notice these signs, it might mean your inner critic is speaking loudly. The good news is that you can learn to quiet it.

2.4 Challenging Negative Self-Talk

The inner critic often thrives on negative self-talk. Negative self-talk is the habit of telling yourself all the things you cannot do, the things that make you feel unworthy, or the reasons you will not succeed. Here is how you can challenge it:

1. **Catch the Thought**: The moment you notice a harsh thought—like "I am not good enough"—stop and label it as negative self-talk.
2. **Question It**: Ask, "Is this thought actually true?" In many cases, you will see it is not based on facts, but on fear or old beliefs.
3. **Replace It**: Come up with a more balanced thought. For example, replace "I will fail at this job" with "I might face challenges, but I can learn as I go." This is not blind positivity; it is a realistic viewpoint that does not limit you.

By repeating this process, you teach your brain to be more forgiving and open-minded.

2.5 How the Inner Critic Affects Confidence

When your inner critic is loud, it can take a big bite out of your confidence. You may feel small or helpless, as if you have no skills or value. Over time, this can lead to:

- **Low Self-Esteem**: You might start believing negative messages, feeling unworthy of good things in life.
- **Anxiety and Stress**: Constantly thinking about your flaws causes tension and worry.
- **Missed Opportunities**: You may skip events, avoid interviews, or shy away from new relationships because you fear you will fail or get hurt.

This is why learning to manage your inner critic is so important. Reducing its power helps you believe in yourself and opens doors to new possibilities.

2.6 The Power of Self-Compassion

One of the best ways to battle the inner critic is through self-compassion. Self-compassion is treating yourself with the same kindness you would give a friend who is struggling. It involves three main parts:

1. **Mindfulness**: Recognizing when you are in pain or when you are being hard on yourself. You step back and notice your thoughts without judgment.
2. **Self-Kindness**: Instead of criticizing yourself, you speak gently. You might say, "It is okay to make mistakes. I am learning."
3. **Common Humanity**: Realizing that everyone makes mistakes and feels inadequate sometimes. You are not alone in your struggles.

When you practice self-compassion, you give yourself room to grow. Instead of blaming yourself for mistakes, you learn from them. Over time, this helps you quiet the inner critic and build a healthier sense of self-worth.

2.7 Practical Techniques to Quiet the Inner Critic

Here are some steps you can take to reduce negative self-talk and increase self-compassion:

1. **Name Your Inner Critic**: Give it a nickname or a character. This helps you see it as separate from your true self. When it pops up, you can say, "Oh, that is just Negative Nancy talking again."
2. **Write It Down**: Journaling can reveal patterns in your self-talk. When you see the same negative statements written over and over, you can challenge them more effectively.

3. **Replace Harsh Words**: Turn "I am so stupid" into "I am learning, and everyone makes mistakes sometimes." Write down alternative statements you can use whenever the inner critic appears.
4. **Use Positive Affirmations**: Short, uplifting phrases can help override negative thoughts. For example: "I am worthy of love and respect." Place these on sticky notes around your home or office.
5. **Seek Support**: Talk to a friend, counselor, or coach. Sharing your feelings can help you see how harsh your inner critic might be. Others can offer a more balanced perspective.
6. **Practice Forgiveness**: Let go of mistakes and past regrets. Remind yourself that you did the best you could at the time. Holding onto guilt only feeds the critic.

2.8 Reframing Failures

Failure is a part of life. Even the most successful people have failed at something. The inner critic often tries to use failures as proof that you are not good enough. But what if you see failure differently?

- **As a Teacher**: Each failure teaches you something. For example, maybe you learned you need better time management or that a certain approach does not work.
- **As a Step Toward Growth**: Every time you fail, you gain experience. That experience can help you do better next time.
- **As Normal**: Everyone fails. When you accept that failure is a normal part of learning, it becomes less scary.

By reframing failure, you take away one of the inner critic's strongest weapons.

2.9 Building Evidence of Your Strengths

A useful way to weaken your inner critic is to gather evidence that shows you are capable. You can do this by:

1. **Making a List of Successes**: Write down your achievements, big or small. This could be academic grades, work projects, or personal victories like overcoming a fear.

2. **Saving Positive Feedback**: Keep an email folder or a physical file of compliments, thank-you notes, or awards. When you feel down, look through them.
3. **Acknowledging Daily Wins**: At the end of each day, note one thing you did well. It might be as small as "I managed to stay calm during an argument" or as large as "I completed a big assignment at work."

Having proof that you are skilled or knowledgeable weakens the critic's claims. It is harder for that negative voice to say, "You are no good," when you have clear examples of your strengths.

2.10 Imagining a Supportive Friend

Sometimes, it helps to imagine what a kind and supportive friend would say to you if she saw you criticizing yourself. She would likely say things like, "You are doing your best," or "I believe in you." You can also imagine saying these kinds of encouraging words to a friend who doubts herself. Notice how gentle and understanding you would be with her. Then, turn that same understanding toward yourself. By shifting your perspective, you become more compassionate in your self-talk.

2.11 Creating a Healthier Inner Voice

Changing your inner critic into a calmer, kinder voice does not happen overnight. However, steady practice makes a big difference. Here is a step-by-step approach you can try:

1. **Observe**: For one or two days, just notice how often you talk negatively to yourself. You might keep a small notebook handy and mark a tally each time.
2. **Identify Triggers**: Look at when your negative self-talk is the worst. Is it when you are under stress at work? Or after you see someone on social media who seems more successful?
3. **Plan**: Before you enter a situation that triggers your inner critic, decide on a few positive or neutral statements you can use to counter the negativity.
4. **Apply**: When negative thoughts pop up, immediately respond with your prepared statements. For instance, if your critic says, "You are going to mess up this presentation," you might respond with, "I have practiced. I am ready, and it is okay if I am not perfect."

5. **Review**: At the end of the day, reflect on how well you handled your inner critic. What worked? What still needs practice?

Over time, you will begin to notice that the negative voice has less power. You will also find that it shows up less frequently or in a weaker form.

2.12 The Link Between the Inner Critic and Stress

When your inner critic is active, it often increases stress. You might feel your heart rate go up or your stomach tighten. You may lose sleep because you keep replaying mistakes in your mind. One way to break this cycle is to use stress-management techniques, such as:

- **Deep Breathing**: Inhale for a count of four, hold for four, and exhale for four.
- **Physical Activity**: Go for a walk, do yoga, or engage in another gentle workout. This can help clear your mind.
- **Mindful Distraction**: Listen to music, read a short story, or do a craft project to shift your focus.

By reducing stress, you also weaken the grip of your inner critic. A calmer mind is more likely to think positively.

2.13 Social Media and the Inner Critic

In today's world, social media can make the inner critic louder. You might see pictures of friends or strangers living what seems like perfect lives, achieving goals easily, or looking flawless in every photo. This can lead you to compare yourself and feel less worthy.

Here are some tips for managing social media comparison:

1. **Limit Your Time Online**: Spend a set amount of time each day on social platforms. Do not scroll endlessly.
2. **Curate Your Feed**: Unfollow or mute accounts that make you feel bad about yourself. Follow accounts that inspire and uplift you instead.
3. **Remember Reality**: People often show only their highlights on social media, not their struggles. Do not assume someone's life is perfect just because their pictures look perfect.

4. **Focus on Your Own Journey**: Remind yourself that everyone's path is different. Celebrate your own progress instead of comparing it to someone else's timeline.

2.14 Practical Exercises to Tame the Inner Critic

1. **The Inner Critic Role-Play**: Pair up with a friend you trust. Ask your friend to pretend to be your inner critic for a moment, saying the things it usually says. Then, respond out loud with positive or balanced statements. This gives you practice standing up for yourself.
2. **Draw Your Inner Critic**: If you like art, draw or paint an image that represents your negative voice. It could be a cloud, a monster, or any symbol. Then, create another drawing that symbolizes self-love or compassion. This exercise helps externalize your thoughts and can make them easier to handle.
3. **Letter of Self-Forgiveness**: Write a letter to yourself, forgiving past mistakes and regrets. Start with, "I forgive myself for..." and be honest. Keep this letter and read it whenever the inner critic tries to shame you about old faults.
4. **Affirmation Recording**: Record yourself saying five positive affirmations on your phone. Play them back each morning and evening, letting your own voice remind you of your worth.

2.15 Knowing When to Seek Professional Help

Sometimes the inner critic can be so loud and persistent that it leads to deep feelings of worthlessness or hopelessness. If you find that your negative self-talk is severely impacting your daily life, it may be time to talk to a professional. A counselor, therapist, or life coach can offer strategies tailored to your needs. There is no shame in seeking help; it can be a powerful step in quieting that inner voice.

2.16 Setting Boundaries With Yourself

Just as we set boundaries with other people, we can set boundaries with our inner critic. You might tell yourself, "I will not engage in negative self-talk before bedtime" or "I will only allow myself to think about past mistakes for 15 minutes, then I will move on." This helps you maintain some control over the *negative messages. It also reminds you that you have the power to decide what thoughts get your attention and how much time you spend on them.*

2.17 The Long-Term Impact of Overcoming the Inner Critic

When you learn to manage and quiet your inner critic, you will likely experience many long-term benefits:

- **Greater Self-Confidence**: You trust yourself more, leading to bolder choices and new achievements.
- **Healthier Emotional Life**: You do not beat yourself up as much, so you feel more calm and balanced.
- **Improved Relationships**: When you treat yourself kindly, you can treat others kindly, too. You also become more open to receiving love and support.

Remember that quieting the inner critic is a journey, not a quick fix. There will be days when the voice is louder than you would like. In those times, be patient and remember all the tools you have learned.

2.18 A Quick Daily Routine to Keep the Critic in Check

- **Morning**: Upon waking, say one positive affirmation. It could be as simple as, "I deserve a good day."
- **Afternoon**: Check in with yourself. If you catch negative thoughts, write them down quickly and replace them with balanced statements.
- **Evening**: List three things you did well today, no matter how small.
- **Before Bed**: Spend a few minutes doing deep breathing or listening to calming music to set your mind at ease.

By following these steps each day, you consistently remind yourself that you are more than the criticisms in your head.

CHAPTER 3

Self-Awareness and Acceptance

3.1 Understanding Self-Awareness

Self-awareness is the ability to look inside yourself and recognize your own feelings, thoughts, and patterns of behavior. It is like turning on a light in a dark room. Once you see what is there, you can navigate more easily. Without self-awareness, it is difficult to understand why you react a certain way or what causes your emotions to rise and fall.

Think of self-awareness as creating a friendly relationship with yourself. You observe your own thoughts and feelings without judging them as "good" or "bad." You become curious about what makes you tick. For example, if you notice your heart beating fast before you speak in a meeting, you might stop and think, "Why am I nervous right now?" Instead of criticizing yourself for feeling that way, you simply explore the reason behind it.

3.2 Why Self-Awareness Matters for Confidence

Confidence often starts with knowing who you are. If you do not understand your own strengths, how can you use them? If you are blind to your weaknesses, how can you improve them? Self-awareness helps you identify both your positive traits and areas where you can grow. This knowledge empowers you to make clear decisions and develop healthy self-esteem.

Some benefits include:

1. **Clarity of Purpose**: When you know what you truly value, it is easier to set goals aligned with those values.
2. **Better Emotional Control**: Recognizing triggers—things that upset or stress you—lets you prepare healthy responses.
3. **Improved Relationships**: Understanding your own habits can help you communicate more openly with others.
4. **Higher Self-Respect**: When you see yourself honestly, you can give yourself credit for your achievements without dismissing them.

3.3 The Difference Between Self-Awareness and Self-Criticism

It is easy to confuse self-awareness with being hard on yourself. In reality, they are quite different:

- **Self-Criticism**: Involves focusing on your flaws in a harsh way. For instance, you might say, "I can never do anything right."
- **Self-Awareness**: Involves noticing areas where you struggle, but viewing them as opportunities to learn. You might say, "I struggle with time management, and I want to find ways to improve."

Self-awareness does not leave you feeling hopeless; instead, it guides you toward solutions. It helps you grow without tearing you down in the process.

3.4 How to Build Self-Awareness

1. **Reflect Daily**: Spend a few minutes each day thinking about how you felt. What made you happy, sad, or frustrated? Writing in a journal can help.
2. **Ask for Feedback**: Friends or family might see patterns you miss. A gentle conversation with someone you trust can offer fresh insights.
3. **Practice Mindfulness**: Take a moment to pause and check in with your body and emotions. Notice tension in your shoulders or butterflies in your stomach. Try to name what you are feeling without judging it.
4. **Notice Your Self-Talk**: Do you often call yourself names like "lazy" or "stupid"? Recognizing negative self-talk is a key step toward breaking that habit.
5. **Use Personality Tools**: Some people find quizzes or self-assessment tools helpful. While they are not always perfect, they can spark new understandings about yourself.

3.5 Embracing Self-Acceptance

Self-acceptance goes hand-in-hand with self-awareness. It means acknowledging all parts of yourself—both positive and negative—and loving yourself anyway. Imagine you have a friend who sometimes makes mistakes but also has wonderful qualities. You do not abandon your friend because of a few flaws. In the same way, you can choose to embrace all aspects of yourself.

Self-acceptance is not about ignoring areas that need improvement. Instead, it is about understanding that you have worth, even if you are not perfect. This mindset can dramatically reduce stress and self-doubt. When you accept yourself, you do not feel trapped by your weaknesses; you simply see them as parts of you that can evolve over time.

3.6 The Cost of Rejecting Yourself

When you refuse to accept who you are, you might experience:

1. **Low Self-Esteem**: Believing you are not good enough can lead to constant self-doubt.
2. **Inner Conflict**: Part of you might want to relax or have fun, but another part insists you have no right to happiness because of your flaws.
3. **Frequent Comparisons**: You may compare yourself to others endlessly, creating jealousy or bitterness.
4. **Strained Relationships**: People who constantly judge themselves often judge others too, causing tension in friendships and family life.

Self-rejection can keep you stuck, while self-acceptance creates room for peace and growth.

3.7 Techniques to Practice Self-Acceptance

1. **Positive Affirmations**: Simple statements like "I am enough" or "I love and accept myself fully" can reprogram negative beliefs.
2. **Gratitude List**: Write down things you appreciate about yourself. For example, "I am kind to my neighbors" or "I have a good sense of humor."
3. **Acknowledge Feelings**: When you feel upset or disappointed, let yourself feel it without pushing it away. This validates your emotions.
4. **Be Kind to Your Body**: Treat yourself with care. This might include getting enough sleep, eating nourishing food, and allowing yourself time to rest.
5. **Focus on Progress, Not Perfection**: Celebrate each small step you take forward, rather than beating yourself up for not being an expert right away.

3.8 Balancing Acceptance and Ambition

Some people worry that if they accept themselves, they might stop trying to improve. But healthy acceptance does not block ambition; it actually supports it. When you accept yourself, you free up mental energy. You no longer waste time hating your flaws or berating yourself. Instead, you focus on solutions and growth.

For example, if you accept that you are not great at public speaking yet, you can calmly look for ways to improve—maybe joining a local speaking club or practicing presentations with friends. On the other hand, if you refuse to accept your shortcoming, you may ignore it, avoid it, or constantly criticize yourself. That cycle of shame can keep you from getting better.

3.9 Self-Awareness in Everyday Life

Self-awareness is not just something you do in your mind. It affects your actions and choices each day:

- **Choosing Your Battles**: When you notice that certain arguments raise your stress without resolving anything, you might decide to walk away or address the issue differently.
- **Handling Triggers**: If you realize you get anxious in crowded places, you can plan ahead. This might involve arriving early or bringing a calming item like a stress ball.
- **Time Management**: By noticing when you feel most energetic or focused, you can schedule important tasks during those periods.
- **Healthy Eating and Exercise**: Recognizing how your body feels after certain foods or workouts can guide you to make better health choices.

3.10 Real-Life Example: Tanya's Insight

Tanya always felt stressed and did not understand why. She began a simple journaling practice. Each evening, she wrote down any strong emotions she felt during the day and what might have caused them. After two weeks, Tanya noticed that she felt extremely anxious whenever she spent too long on social media before bed. Reading about other people's successes made her feel like she was not doing enough with her own life. With this new self-awareness, Tanya decided to set a limit on her nighttime scrolling. Over time, she felt calmer and more confident. By being aware of the trigger, she could take action to protect her mental well-being.

3.11 Building Emotional Awareness

Emotions are powerful, and they can direct our actions if we are not careful. Building emotional awareness means recognizing what you are feeling and why. Some tips:

1. **Name the Emotion**: Is it sadness, excitement, anger, or fear? Labeling it can help you understand what is happening.
2. **Check the Intensity**: Rate how strong the feeling is on a scale of 1 to 10. This helps you measure how urgent it is to deal with it.
3. **Notice Physical Signs**: Emotions often show up in your body. For instance, a fast heartbeat might indicate anxiety; tight shoulders could mean stress.
4. **Pause Before Reacting**: If you feel angry, take a slow breath before speaking. This gives you time to respond wisely instead of lashing out.

As you become more aware of your emotional states, you can keep them from overpowering your better judgment. This leads to calmer, more confident decision-making.

3.12 Acceptance of Past Mistakes

Self-acceptance includes forgiving yourself for things you did in the past. Everyone makes mistakes. Holding onto guilt or shame does not fix what happened; it only drains your energy. You can try:

- **Writing a Forgiveness Letter**: Address it to yourself, acknowledging the mistake and stating that you choose to let go of the guilt.
- **Making Amends**: If possible, apologize or fix the situation. If it is not possible, focus on learning the lesson for the future.
- **Learning the Lesson**: Ask, "What can I learn from this mistake so I do not repeat it?"

By accepting past errors, you open a door to personal healing. You also strengthen your belief in your ability to grow and change.

3.13 Social Influences on Self-Awareness

Humans are social creatures. The people around us can help—or hinder—our self-awareness. Consider how:

1. **Family Beliefs**: Values you learned at home might shape your sense of self. Identify which ones still fit your life and which ones you want to rethink.
2. **Cultural Norms**: In some cultures, being shy might be seen as polite, while in others, being outspoken is praised. Understanding cultural expectations can help you see where certain feelings come from.
3. **Peer Groups**: Friends can provide honest opinions about your behavior. The key is to choose friends who genuinely want to support your growth.

3.14 Using Mindful Practices for Self-Awareness

Mindfulness is about staying present in the moment. Simple mindfulness exercises can increase your self-awareness:

1. **Breathing Exercise**: Close your eyes and pay attention to your breath for one minute. Notice the inhale, the exhale, and how your body feels.
2. **Body Scan**: Mentally scan your body from head to toe, noticing tension or relaxation.
3. **Mindful Eating**: Take a small bite of food. Chew slowly, noticing the taste and texture. This practice teaches you to observe details you might usually overlook.
4. **Walking Meditation**: Walk slowly, focusing on each step and how your feet connect with the ground.

These activities train you to notice subtle details in your thoughts and feelings, boosting self-awareness.

3.15 Setting Personal Boundaries Through Self-Awareness

When you know your limits, you can set healthier boundaries. For instance, you might realize you feel overwhelmed by too many social events in a single week. That awareness can prompt you to block out alone time in your schedule. Or maybe you notice you feel uneasy when a coworker frequently complains to you. Recognizing that discomfort can lead you to gently tell them you need to limit negative talk.

Boundaries protect your energy and well-being. By being self-aware, you spot problems earlier and address them in kinder, calmer ways.

3.16 How Acceptance Affects Your Mental Health

Accepting yourself, including your struggles, can lower stress and anxiety. You stop beating yourself up over issues, which removes a huge mental burden. For instance, if you have a health challenge like diabetes or an anxiety disorder, accepting that it is part of your life allows you to focus on effective management rather than denial or shame. In turn, this acceptance can help you find solutions and support that truly benefit you.

3.17 Self-Acceptance Versus Settling

Be careful not to mistake self-acceptance for "settling" in an unhealthy situation. Accepting yourself means understanding you are worthy of love and respect. It does not mean you have to tolerate a toxic workplace, an abusive relationship, or any environment that harms you. Rather, true self-acceptance often gives you the courage to leave situations that do not align with your well-being. You realize you deserve better and become motivated to seek healthier surroundings.

3.18 Action Steps to Grow Self-Awareness and Acceptance

Here is a quick plan to help you stay on track:

1. **Create a Self-Check Routine**: Pick one time a day to pause and ask, "How am I feeling right now?"
2. **Use a Journal**: Write about what triggers strong emotions. Note any patterns or recurring themes.
3. **Practice Gratitude**: Each evening, list three things you are thankful for about yourself. It could be a skill, a moment of kindness, or something new you learned.
4. **Share With a Friend or Mentor**: A quick chat can provide feedback and encouragement as you grow.

5. **Celebrate Progress**: Maybe you used to ignore your feelings. Now you notice them more quickly. That is a big step! Recognize and value your improvements.

3.19 A Short Visualization Exercise

Try this short activity:

1. **Close Your Eyes**: *Take a slow breath in, then out.*
2. **Picture Your Ideal Self**: *Imagine you at your most content and confident. How do you stand? How do you speak to yourself? What do you spend time on?*
3. **Embrace Imperfections**: *Notice any "flaws" or worries that come up in the image. Gently include them, realizing you are lovable even with these imperfections.*
4. **Return to Reality**: *Open your eyes. Write down what you saw or felt. Keep these notes as a reminder of your goals and your worth.*

CHAPTER 4

Setting Goals and Building Motivation

4.1 Why Goals Matter

Goals are like a roadmap for your life. They give you something to aim for and can provide a sense of direction and purpose. Without goals, it is easy to feel lost or stuck, unsure of what to do next. With clear goals, you can measure your progress, celebrate victories, and adjust when things change.

Think of setting goals as deciding on a destination. If you do not choose where you want to go, you will wander around aimlessly. But once you have a target, you can plan how to get there, step by step. Goals help you live your life more intentionally, making it easier to see that your actions matter.

4.2 Connecting Goals to Your Values

A goal is more powerful when it aligns with your core values. For instance, if one of your values is helping people, setting a goal to volunteer or mentor might feel especially meaningful. On the other hand, if you chase a goal that goes against your values, you might lose motivation quickly.

Start by listing your top five values, such as family, creativity, independence, honesty, or health. Then, consider which goals support these values. For example, if family is important to you, a goal might be to spend dedicated time each week with your children or parents. This connection between values and goals will fuel your motivation and help you stay committed.

4.3 Different Types of Goals

1. **Short-Term Goals**: These can be achieved relatively quickly, sometimes in a week or a few months. For example, cleaning out a closet or finishing a short training course.
2. **Medium-Term Goals**: These take a bit longer, perhaps six months to a year. You might aim to improve your public speaking skills or save a certain amount of money.

3. **Long-Term Goals**: These can span years, like earning a degree, purchasing a home, or starting a business. They require consistent effort and planning.

Having a mix of short, medium, and long-term goals ensures you have frequent wins (short-term) while still aiming for bigger achievements down the road (long-term).

4.4 Setting S.M.A.R.T. Goals

A common framework for effective goal setting is S.M.A.R.T.:

- **Specific**: Make your goal clear and detailed. Instead of saying, "I want to get fit," say, "I want to run 3 miles without stopping."
- **Measurable**: You should be able to track progress. For instance, the distance you can run or the number of times you exercise per week.
- **Achievable**: Your goal should be challenging but still within reach. If it is too extreme, you risk feeling discouraged.
- **Relevant**: Tie the goal to something that matters to you and your values.
- **Time-Bound**: Set a deadline or time frame to help motivate you. For example, "I will run 3 miles without stopping by the end of three months."

Using the S.M.A.R.T. method forces you to be clear about what you want and how you plan to get it.

4.5 Overcoming Obstacles to Goal-Setting

Some people hesitate to set goals because they fear failure or are unsure where to start. Common obstacles include:

1. **Fear of Failure**: You might avoid setting a goal because you worry you will not succeed. However, remember that failure can teach important lessons and is often a stepping stone to success.
2. **Lack of Clarity**: If you do not know what you truly want, it is hard to set a meaningful goal. In this case, spend time exploring your interests and values.
3. **Overwhelming Goals**: Sometimes goals feel too big. Break them down into smaller, manageable tasks.

4. **Procrastination**: Delaying action can kill motivation. Create mini-deadlines and small steps to get started and keep momentum.

Recognizing these obstacles early can help you plan ways to work around them.

4.6 Finding Your Motivation

Motivation is the inner drive that pushes you to take action. It can come from many places:

1. **Internal Desire**: You pursue something because it excites or fulfills you. This is often called intrinsic motivation.
2. **External Rewards**: You work toward a goal for an external prize, such as money, recognition, or status. This is extrinsic motivation.
3. **Social Influence**: Sometimes the encouragement or competition from friends and family can spark motivation.

Ideally, you want a strong internal desire for your goal, because that will keep you going even when external rewards or praise are missing.

4.7 Practical Steps to Stay Motivated

1. **Write Down Your Goals**: Seeing them on paper or a digital planner helps remind you of your commitments.
2. **Visualize Success**: Spend a minute each day picturing yourself achieving the goal. How do you feel? What do you see? This mental rehearsal can boost your drive.
3. **Break It Down**: Slice big goals into smaller tasks. Each completed task gives you a sense of achievement, fueling further motivation.
4. **Track Your Progress**: Keep a record of what you have done. This could be a chart or a simple checklist. Watching your progress grow is motivating.
5. **Reward Yourself**: Plan small rewards for hitting milestones. It could be a special meal, a short trip, or even a new book you have been wanting to read.

4.8 Maintaining Momentum

It is common to start off very excited about a goal, then lose steam over time. Life gets busy, or the initial thrill fades. Here are ways to keep momentum:

- **Schedule Regular Check-Ins**: Set a time each week or month to review your progress. This keeps your goal at the forefront of your mind.
- **Adjust as Needed**: If something is not working, do not give up. Change your plan. Maybe you need more resources, different techniques, or a simpler first step.
- **Stay Inspired**: Read articles, watch videos, or follow people who have achieved similar goals. Their stories can rekindle your own fire.
- **Surround Yourself with Positive People**: Spend time with individuals who encourage you. Their energy can help you push forward when you feel tired.

4.9 Dealing with Setbacks

No matter how well you plan, setbacks will happen. You might get sick, face financial problems, or lose motivation. Instead of seeing these setbacks as the end, view them as temporary roadblocks. Ask yourself:

1. **What Can I Learn?** A setback can show you areas that need attention. Maybe you need better time management or more realistic deadlines.
2. **Who Can Help Me?** Friends, mentors, or professionals might have ideas to help you recover quickly.
3. **How Can I Adjust My Goal?** You might extend the deadline or break down the goal further so it is still achievable.

Learning to bounce back from setbacks is part of growing your overall confidence.

4.10 Celebrating Small Wins

Many people wait to celebrate until they have reached the end goal. But celebrating small victories along the way can keep you motivated. For instance, if your goal is to write a 50-page report, celebrate after every five pages. These little boosts of joy remind you that progress is happening, and it is worth recognizing.

Celebrations do not need to be expensive or grand. They can be as simple as giving yourself a break to listen to music you love, enjoying a treat, or sharing your accomplishment with a friend.

4.11 Balancing Multiple Goals

At times, you may have more than one goal. Perhaps you want to advance in your career, improve your fitness, and learn a new language all at once. While it is good to be ambitious, juggling multiple goals can lead to burnout if not managed well. Here are some tips:

1. **Prioritize**: Decide which goal is most urgent or meaningful right now. Focus on that first while keeping the others at a slower pace.
2. **Create a Timeline**: You might allocate certain months for specific goals. For example, focus on career improvement for the first three months, then add in fitness in the next three months.
3. **Stay Realistic**: Check in with your schedule, energy, and resources. Do not pile on so many goals that you end up not making progress on any of them.
4. **Evaluate Often**: Every month, see what is working and what is not. Adjust your plans so you do not lose motivation.

4.12 The Role of Accountability

Having someone to hold you accountable can be a powerful motivator. This could be a friend, family member, or a coach who checks in on your progress. You might:

- Schedule weekly calls or messages to share updates.
- Promise to show your completed tasks to this person by a certain date.
- Create a mini competition with a friend who has a similar goal.

Accountability helps ensure you do not push your goals to the bottom of your to-do list. It is a gentle nudge that reminds you people are supporting your efforts and waiting to hear about your progress.

4.13 How Motivation Affects Confidence

When you work steadily toward a goal and see yourself making progress, your confidence naturally grows. Each success, no matter how small, proves you can set a target and move closer to it. That sense of achievement makes you more likely to believe in your abilities in other areas of life too.

Motivation is like fuel in a car. Without it, even the best engine (or the most capable person) will not get very far. But when you have motivation, you have the energy to keep going, to overcome roadblocks, and to eventually reach your destination.

4.14 Self-Care and Goal Pursuit

It can be tempting to push yourself too hard when you are motivated. Some people skip meals, lose sleep, or neglect relationships in the name of their goals. However, self-care is essential if you want to maintain long-term motivation. Proper rest, exercise, and leisure activities help keep your mind and body in good shape, making you more effective when you do work toward your goals.

If you notice you are feeling drained or resentful about your goal, it might be time to step back. Evaluate whether you are sacrificing too much. Often, adding short breaks or fun activities back into your routine can refresh your energy and creativity.

4.15 Real-Life Example: Maria's Career Leap

Maria wanted to switch from a customer service job to a position in marketing. She set a long-term goal: "Land a marketing coordinator role by next year." She then broke it down:

1. **Short-Term Goal**: *Research and choose an online marketing course (done in two weeks).*
2. **Medium-Term Goal**: *Complete the course and build a personal portfolio (within three months).*
3. **Long-Term Goal**: *Apply for coordinator roles (after building enough skills and examples of her work).*

Maria stayed motivated by watching marketing tutorials and connecting with people in that field. Whenever she finished a section of the online course, she treated herself to a nice dinner. Although she faced setbacks—like struggling with certain course modules—she adjusted her plan rather than giving up. After several months, Maria felt confident enough to send out applications. Eventually, she secured the marketing coordinator role she had aimed for. This experience strengthened her confidence because she saw firsthand that careful goal-setting and persistent motivation can pay off.

4.16 Handling Criticism and Doubt

When you set ambitious goals, you might face criticism from others or even internal doubt. Some people might say your goal is unrealistic, or you might worry you are not capable. In these moments:

1. **Remember Your Why**: Revisit the reasons you chose this goal. Does it align with your values? Does it excite you?
2. **Seek Support**: Talk to friends or mentors who believe in you. Sometimes a few encouraging words can counteract negativity.
3. **Reframe Doubt**: Doubt can be a sign you are pushing beyond your comfort zone, which is often where real growth happens.

Criticism can also be a chance to learn. Some feedback might be useful. You can evaluate whether there is truth in it and adapt your plan. But do not let purely negative or mocking remarks derail you.

4.17 Tools and Resources for Goal-Setting

Technology can simplify and support your goal-setting process. Consider:

- **Apps**: Many free or low-cost apps help track habits or progress (e.g., Habitica, Strides, or Todoist).
- **Calendars**: A physical or digital calendar can keep you aware of deadlines.
- **Vision Boards**: Some people create a collage of images, words, or quotes that represent their goals. Keeping it somewhere visible serves as a daily reminder.
- **Online Communities**: Forums or social media groups for people with similar goals can provide tips, moral support, and advice.

4.18 Checking for Progress and Adjusting

Regularly reviewing your goals is a vital part of maintaining motivation. You can do a monthly or quarterly review where you ask:

1. **What progress have I made?**
2. **What challenges or delays came up?**
3. **Do I need to change my strategy or timeline?**
4. **Do these goals still reflect my values?**

If your goal no longer feels relevant or exciting, it might be time to refine it or replace it with a more suitable target. Changing goals is not failure; it is a natural response to new information or shifting priorities.

4.19 Celebrating the Journey, Not Just the Destination

Remember that achieving goals is not just about the finish line. Much of the growth happens during the journey. You learn new skills, develop resilience, and expand your sense of possibility. Even if you do not achieve the exact result you aimed for, the process itself can teach you important lessons, which ultimately builds your confidence.

Appreciate every stage of the process. When you look back, you will see how far you have come, and that in itself is an accomplishment.

CHAPTER 5

Self-Care for Mental and Emotional Health

5.1 What Is Self-Care?

Self-care is the practice of looking after your own mental and emotional well-being. Sometimes, people think self-care is selfish. But it is actually very helpful, not only for you but also for those around you. When you feel calm and stable, you can handle your responsibilities better. You can also be kinder and more supportive to other people in your life.

Self-care can include many activities: taking a short walk, journaling about your day, enjoying a hobby, or simply setting aside a few minutes to breathe deeply. Each person's version of self-care might look different. The key is to find what makes you feel better mentally and emotionally.

5.2 Why Self-Care Matters for Women

Women often wear many hats. Some are caregivers, professionals, partners, friends, and more—sometimes all at once. Because of these roles, women can feel pressure to take care of everyone else before themselves. Over time, this can lead to burnout, stress, and exhaustion. You might feel guilty if you pause to rest or relax. However, self-care is not a luxury. It is a way to recharge so that you can keep giving your best to the people and tasks that matter to you.

When you care for your mental and emotional health, you also show others that rest and balance are important. You become an example of healthy behavior for friends, family members, and even coworkers. They learn that it is okay to slow down sometimes and pay attention to personal needs.

5.3 Signs You Need More Self-Care

It can be easy to get so busy that you do not notice you are running on empty. Here are some signs that you might need to focus on self-care:

1. **Constant Tiredness**: Even after a full night's sleep, you still feel drained or exhausted.
2. **Mood Swings**: Small problems make you very upset, or you feel irritated more often than usual.
3. **Lack of Interest**: Activities you once enjoyed now seem boring or overwhelming.
4. **Physical Symptoms**: Headaches, tight muscles, or frequent illnesses can appear when stress is high.
5. **Trouble Sleeping**: You cannot fall asleep, or you wake up multiple times at night with worrying thoughts.

Noticing these signs is not meant to scare you. Instead, it is a call to action: slow down and give yourself the care you deserve.

5.4 The Connection Between Mental and Emotional Health

Mental health involves your overall psychological well-being—how you think, feel, and behave. Emotional health is a part of this, focusing on your ability to handle and express emotions in a healthy way. While they are closely linked, you can think of mental health as the big umbrella and emotional health as one part of it.

A strong mental and emotional state helps you:

- **Cope with Stress**: You can manage the ups and downs of life without feeling constantly overwhelmed.
- **Form Healthy Relationships**: You can communicate your feelings and needs, and also listen to others without getting overly defensive or anxious.
- **Make Clear Decisions**: It is easier to solve problems and plan for the future when your mind is not burdened by heavy stress or unresolved feelings.

5.5 Physical Health as Part of Self-Care

Although we are focusing on mental and emotional well-being, it is important to note that physical health has a huge impact on how you feel inside. Here are some physical habits that can improve your mental state:

1. **Regular Exercise**: You do not have to become a marathon runner. Even short, brisk walks or simple stretches can help your brain produce endorphins—chemicals that lift your mood.
2. **Proper Rest**: Aim for 7-9 hours of sleep per night. Good sleep restores both your body and mind.
3. **Balanced Nutrition**: Eating a variety of fruits, vegetables, whole grains, and proteins supports your mood and energy levels.
4. **Hydration**: Staying hydrated helps you think clearly and feel more alert.

While these might sound like basics, they are powerful parts of any self-care routine.

5.6 Daily Habits for Emotional Well-Being

Taking care of your emotions can be done in small daily steps. Here are a few practices you can build into your routine:

1. **Gratitude Journaling**: Write down at least one thing you are thankful for each day. This trains your mind to notice positives rather than only problems.
2. **Set Boundaries on Media**: Constantly consuming negative news or scrolling through social media can drain you. Limit your screen time, especially if it makes you anxious or upset.
3. **Breathing Exercises**: Take a few slow, deep breaths when you wake up or before a stressful meeting. Focus on how the air feels entering and leaving your body.
4. **Mindful Moments**: While brushing your teeth or washing dishes, pay attention to the experience instead of letting your thoughts race. Being present can calm your mind.
5. **Talk It Out**: If something is bothering you, share it with a trusted friend or family member. Sometimes, speaking your worries out loud helps you see solutions more clearly.

5.7 Creating a Self-Care Plan

It can help to have a written or mental plan for how you will take care of yourself each day or week. Think of it like a checklist. You might decide:

- **Morning Routine**: 5 minutes of quiet reflection or gentle stretching.

- **Afternoon Break**: A short walk outside or a quick journaling session.
- **Evening Wind-Down**: Reading a book you enjoy, drinking a calming tea, or doing a breathing exercise before bed.

You can tweak this plan to fit your schedule. The main point is to include regular moments for rest and reflection. If you do not plan for self-care, it is easy for it to be pushed aside by other demands.

5.8 Emotional Release Activities

Sometimes, stress or anger can build up, and it feels like a pressure cooker inside your mind. Finding ways to safely release these feelings can prevent them from overflowing in harmful ways:

1. **Creative Expression**: Painting, drawing, coloring, or writing poetry can help you process strong emotions.
2. **Physical Release**: Dancing, running, or even punching a pillow can help let out tension stored in your body.
3. **Crying**: There is no shame in shedding tears if you feel overwhelmed. Crying is a natural way for the body to release built-up emotion.
4. **Talking to a Counselor**: A therapist or counselor can guide you through deeper emotional processing, especially if you feel stuck.

Releasing emotions in a healthy way helps you regain balance and prevents negativity from building up.

5.9 The Role of Relaxation Techniques

Relaxation techniques are specific methods designed to reduce stress and calm your mind. Some common ones include:

- **Progressive Muscle Relaxation (PMR)**: You tense and then relax each muscle group in your body, usually starting with your toes and moving up to your head.
- **Guided Imagery**: You listen to or imagine a peaceful scene, focusing on the details, like the sound of waves or the feel of grass under your feet.
- **Meditation**: Sitting in a quiet place, you focus on your breath or a repeated word (mantra). When thoughts drift, you gently bring your focus back.

These techniques do not take much time. Even 5-10 minutes can make a difference in how you feel throughout the day.

5.10 Dealing with Stressful Situations

Life will always bring some level of stress. Whether it is a tight work deadline or a family issue, you cannot eliminate every source of worry. What you can do is change how you respond:

1. **Identify What You Can Control**: Write down your worries. Circle the ones you can do something about, and let go of those you cannot.
2. **Break Tasks into Steps**: A big challenge can feel crushing, but breaking it into smaller tasks can reduce overwhelm.
3. **Take Short Breaks**: Work for a while, then pause for a mental reset. Your mind needs little rests just like your body does.
4. **Ask for Help**: Talk to someone who might have been in your situation or who can offer support. There is no shame in seeking help.

These strategies ensure you are not just pushing stress down where it can grow bigger, but rather managing it in healthy ways.

5.11 Social Connections and Emotional Support

Though self-care often focuses on you, it is also important to remember that humans are social beings. Spending quality time with people who care about you can fill your emotional tank. A supportive conversation can be a form of self-care as well. You might:

- **Reach Out to a Friend**: Send a text or make a call to share what is going on in your life.
- **Join a Community Group**: Look for clubs or groups that share your interests, whether it is a book club or a walking group.
- **Volunteer**: Helping others can boost your mood and give you a sense of purpose.
- **Plan Get-Togethers**: Even a quick coffee date can brighten your day.

Remember, a healthy support system is part of caring for your emotional needs.

5.12 Managing Negative Self-Talk Through Self-Care

Negative self-talk can be a big drain on your emotional health. Self-care includes monitoring your internal dialogue. Here are some ways to handle negative thoughts when they pop up:

1. **Pause and Identify**: Notice the negative thought, then label it: "Here is that voice telling me I am not good enough."
2. **Replace It with Kindness**: Talk to yourself like you would talk to a good friend. For example, say, "I might not have all the answers, but I am doing my best."
3. **Use a Mantra**: Short phrases like "I am learning," or "I am worthy of care," can remind you to treat yourself with compassion.

Over time, these small shifts in thought can greatly improve your emotional well-being.

5.13 Myths About Self-Care

1. **Myth**: "Self-care is only about spa days or massages."
   Reality: While treating yourself can be part of self-care, it is also about daily habits that keep you balanced, like getting enough sleep or talking kindly to yourself.
2. **Myth**: "Self-care is selfish."
   Reality: Caring for your mental and emotional health makes you better able to support others. It is a win-win situation.
3. **Myth**: "I have no time for self-care."
   Reality: Even five minutes of quiet breathing can help you reset. It is about making small spaces in your day, not finding huge chunks of free time.
4. **Myth**: "Self-care fixes everything instantly."
   Reality: Self-care is a practice. It does not erase all problems overnight, but it helps you handle them with a steadier mind.

5.14 Balancing Responsibilities and Self-Care

For many women, life is a juggling act. You might be looking after children, working long hours, or helping an elderly parent. You might wonder, "How can I take care of myself when so many people depend on me?" The truth is, when you are running on empty, you will not be able to help others as effectively. Sometimes, delegating tasks or saying "no" to extra obligations is necessary to protect your mental space.

- **Delegating**: If your kids are old enough, let them do simple chores. If you live with a partner, share tasks.
- **Setting Boundaries**: If someone asks you to handle something you truly do not have time for, it is okay to say no.
- **Using Short Breaks Wisely**: A 10-minute rest might not sound like much, but it can recharge your energy.

5.15 Finding Joy in Everyday Activities

Self-care does not always mean adding new tasks. Sometimes, it is about finding pleasure in what you already do. For example:

- **Mindful Eating**: Instead of rushing through lunch, really taste each bite. Notice the flavors and textures.
- **Listening to Music**: Play your favorite songs while doing chores. Music can lift your mood and make daily tasks more pleasant.
- **Simple Rewards**: After finishing a challenging task, treat yourself to something small like a piece of dark chocolate or a few minutes of reading.

By turning everyday moments into positive experiences, you fill your day with little boosts of happiness.

5.16 Tips for Emotional First Aid

Just as you have a first aid kit for physical injuries, it helps to have a plan for emotional emergencies, such as:

1. **A Comforting Playlist**: Songs that make you feel safe or understood.
2. **Contact List**: Names and numbers of close friends or family who can offer support.
3. **Positive Notes**: Messages written by you or loved ones that remind you of your strengths.
4. **Grounding Object**: A small item (like a pebble or keychain) you can hold to remind yourself of the present moment when anxiety strikes.

Having these ready can help you cope when strong emotions hit unexpectedly.

5.17 The Importance of Professional Help

Sometimes, personal efforts are not enough to manage ongoing mental or emotional challenges. If you find that low mood, anxiety, or stress is interfering with your daily life, talking to a mental health professional can be a big step forward. Therapists and counselors are trained to help you navigate tough feelings, break unhelpful patterns, and find healthier ways to cope.

Seeking help is a form of self-care. It shows courage and responsibility, not weakness. Many people benefit from therapy sessions, group support, or even online counseling platforms.

5.18 Self-Care for Specific Life Challenges

- **Chronic Illness**: *Living with a long-term health condition can be stressful. Self-care might include more rest, gentle stretches, or setting clear limits on your daily activities.*
- **Motherhood**: *The demands of caring for children can be overwhelming. A few quiet moments of "me time," even if it is just locking the bathroom door for a short break, can work wonders.*
- **High-Stress Jobs**: *If your job is very demanding, schedule mini-breaks during the day and longer time off whenever possible to avoid burnout.*
- **Grief and Loss**: *Self-care might involve allowing yourself time to cry, talking with a grief counselor, or honoring the memory of a loved one in a meaningful way.*

In each case, the basic principles of self-care—rest, emotional processing, and seeking help—still apply. You may just need to adapt them to your unique situation.

CHAPTER 6

Healthy Boundaries and Assertiveness

6.1 What Are Boundaries?

Boundaries are the invisible lines that define how you allow others to treat you and how you treat them. They help protect your emotional space and personal well-being. Think of boundaries as a fence around a home. A fence does not mean you hate your neighbors; it simply shows where your property begins and theirs ends. In relationships, boundaries let other people know what is acceptable and what is not.

Healthy boundaries help you express your needs, feelings, and limits in a respectful manner. They also allow you to show respect for the other person's boundaries. Without boundaries, you may feel taken advantage of or overwhelmed by others' demands.

6.2 Why Do Women Often Struggle with Boundaries?

Many women are taught to be nurturing, polite, and helpful from an early age. While these qualities are positive, they can sometimes lead women to say "yes" when they really mean "no." They might worry about appearing rude or unkind if they set limits.

Society also often praises women for self-sacrifice, labeling them as "good" daughters, mothers, or workers when they put others first. This pressure can make it difficult to assert personal needs. Yet, constantly ignoring your own limits can lead to resentment, stress, and burnout.

6.3 Assertiveness: A Key Part of Setting Boundaries

Assertiveness is the ability to express your feelings, needs, and rights calmly and honestly, without stepping on other people's rights. It falls in the middle of two extremes:

- **Passive Behavior**: You do not speak up for yourself. You let others dictate decisions or walk over your needs. You might feel unheard or resentful.
- **Aggressive Behavior**: You express your needs forcefully, without considering others' feelings. You might appear threatening or rude.

Assertiveness is about balance: respecting your own needs while also respecting the rights of others. This style of communication helps create clear, healthy relationships.

6.4 Common Fears About Being Assertive

Some women hesitate to be assertive due to various fears:

1. **Fear of Conflict**: Worrying that voicing a boundary will lead to an argument.
2. **Fear of Rejection**: Thinking people will dislike you if you say "no" or stand up for yourself.
3. **Fear of Being Seen as Mean**: Concern that people will label you as rude or selfish.
4. **Fear of Losing Relationships**: Anxiety that friends or family will leave if you set limits.

Understanding these fears can help you address them head-on. Assertiveness, when done kindly, often leads to healthier relationships in the long run because both parties feel respected.

6.5 Types of Boundaries

Here are some main types of boundaries you might need to consider in your life:

1. **Emotional Boundaries**: Protecting your feelings and emotional well-being. For example, saying you are not comfortable discussing certain personal topics.
2. **Physical Boundaries**: Referring to your personal space and body. This can mean telling someone not to touch you in a certain way or needing space when feeling overwhelmed.

3. **Time Boundaries**: Guarding how you spend your time. This might involve declining extra tasks when your schedule is full or not answering work emails after certain hours.
4. **Material Boundaries**: Involving your belongings or finances. For instance, deciding who can borrow your car and under what conditions.
5. **Mental Boundaries**: Respecting and honoring your own thoughts and opinions. You do not allow others to belittle or dismiss your perspective.

Every person has different comfort levels, so boundaries can vary widely. Knowing which areas you feel most uncomfortable or stressed about can guide you in setting clearer limits.

6.6 Recognizing When Boundaries Are Weak

You might notice certain signs that show your boundaries need strengthening:

- **Constant Resentment**: You feel annoyed or angry at people for asking too much of you, even if you do not say anything out loud.
- **Feeling Overwhelmed**: Your schedule is packed with commitments you did not really want to accept.
- **Difficulty Saying No**: You often say "yes" to requests, then regret it later.
- **Emotional Exhaustion**: You feel drained after interacting with certain people who do not respect your limits.
- **Guilt**: You experience guilt for even thinking about putting your own needs first.

These feelings are signals that you might need to practice setting stronger boundaries.

6.7 How to Begin Setting Boundaries

1. **Identify Your Limits**: Take a moment to figure out what makes you uncomfortable or stressed. Do you dislike last-minute changes to plans? Does it bother you when a friend always borrows money and does not repay? Write these down.

2. **Be Clear and Direct**: When you set a boundary, you must communicate it openly. For example, say, "I can only stay for one hour," or "I need a heads-up before you come over."
3. **Stay Calm**: Express your boundary in a friendly, but firm tone. Anger or aggression can make the other person defensive.
4. **Offer a Brief Explanation (If Needed)**: You do not owe everyone a long reason, but a short explanation can help them understand. "I am not free on Saturdays because that is my family day."
5. **Avoid Over-Apologizing**: You have the right to set boundaries without feeling guilty. Apologizing too much can weaken your message.

6.8 Communicating Assertively

When talking about boundaries, try using "I" statements. This focuses on your feelings rather than blaming the other person. For example:

- **Aggressive**: "You always ignore my schedule and never care about my time!"
- **Assertive**: "I feel stressed when plans change without notice. I need a warning at least one day in advance."

The second statement is clearer and less likely to spark a fight. You are simply stating how you feel and what you need.

6.9 Dealing with Pushback

Sometimes, people react negatively when you first set boundaries, especially if they have become used to you always saying "yes." They might:

- **Complain or Whine**: "You used to be so flexible; why are you being difficult now?"
- **Act Hurt**: "I can't believe you won't help me this time. I thought we were friends."
- **Try to Guilt Trip**: "I guess I will just have to manage on my own since you do not care."

It can be challenging to stand your ground, but remember that you are not responsible for other people's emotional responses. Reassure them (if you wish) that you still value the relationship, but you also need to take care of yourself. Often, people will adjust over time if you remain consistent.

6.10 Setting Boundaries at Work

Work can be a place where boundaries blur, especially if you want to prove yourself. You might overwork, check emails at all hours, or take on tasks that are not part of your job. Over time, this can lead to burnout. To protect your mental health and professional performance:

1. **Clarify Your Role**: Understand what your duties are and politely refuse tasks that fall far outside them if you are already swamped.
2. **Manage Your Availability**: If possible, avoid replying to emails late at night or on weekends unless it is an emergency.
3. **Use Your Breaks**: Take your lunch or short breaks to rest or walk around, instead of working straight through.
4. **Speak Up Early**: If a deadline is unreasonable, say so. Offer solutions: "I can finish this by Friday if I do not have to handle Task X until Monday."

Being assertive at work can increase respect from your colleagues, as they see you know your limits and stand by them.

6.11 Boundaries in Friendships

Friendships are supposed to be supportive, but even good friends can push boundaries if they do not know where your comfort zone ends. Maybe a friend drops by unannounced or shares personal details about you with others. Here is how you can handle it:

- **Gently Explain**: "I enjoy your visits, but I need at least a text or call before you come over."
- **Request Privacy**: "I appreciate your curiosity, but I would rather keep this information between us."
- **Offer Alternatives**: If your friend wants to hang out more than you can handle, say, "I can't meet tonight, but I am free on Saturday."

True friends will try to respect your boundaries once you make them clear.

6.12 Boundaries in Family Relationships

Family members often feel they have a right to comment on or interfere in each other's lives. While family ties can be strong, you still have the right to set limits. For example:

- **Parents**: They might expect you to be available for every gathering. You can say, "I can stay for two hours, but then I have other plans."
- **Siblings**: A brother or sister might tease you about your choices. You can respond, "I understand you have an opinion, but I need you to stop making fun of me."
- **Extended Family**: Relatives might pry into your personal life. A short, polite reply like "I prefer not to talk about that" is enough.

It can feel harder to set boundaries with family, but it is still necessary for your emotional well-being.

6.13 Overcoming Guilt

Feeling guilty when you set boundaries is common, especially if you have rarely done it before. Remind yourself:

- You have the right to protect your mental and emotional health.
- Saying "no" does not mean you do not care—it means you are one person who cannot do everything.
- People who truly respect you will respect your limits.
- Guilt often happens because you are used to over-giving. Give yourself time to adjust to a healthier balance.

You can also talk to a friend or counselor about these guilty feelings. Sometimes, hearing that it is okay from someone else can help you believe it for yourself.

6.14 Assertiveness vs. Aggression in Practice

Let us look at a clear scenario:

- **Scenario**: Your coworker frequently criticizes your work in a sarcastic tone. It is affecting your confidence and mood.

- **Passive Response**: You say nothing and let the coworker keep doing it. You might feel hurt and angry inside, but you try to ignore it.
- **Aggressive Response**: You shout at them, "Shut up! You are the worst person in this office!" This could harm your professional image and escalate conflict.
- **Assertive Response**: You approach them privately and say, "I find your remarks hurtful. I am open to constructive feedback, but the sarcastic tone makes me uncomfortable. I would appreciate if you could talk to me about any concerns more respectfully."

In the assertive response, you address the problem directly without attacking the other person's character. This style promotes healthier communication.

6.15 The Power of Saying "No"

"No" is a complete sentence, though it may feel uncomfortable to say. You can soften it if you like, but you do not need to give excuses. For instance:

- "No, I can't commit to that right now."
- "No, that does not work for me."
- "I need to say no this time."

You might add a brief explanation if you want, like "I already have too much on my plate." But do not feel pressured to offer a detailed account. Practicing saying "no" in small ways can build your confidence for bigger situations.

6.16 When Boundaries Are Violated

Despite your best efforts, some people might ignore your boundaries. This can be hurtful and frustrating. If someone repeatedly disrespects your limits, you may need to:

1. **Reinforce the Boundary**: Calmly remind them again: "I have told you before that I am not comfortable with this."
2. **State Consequences**: If they continue, explain what you will do. For example, "If you keep talking about this topic, I will have to end the conversation."
3. **Follow Through**: If they still do not stop, end the phone call or leave the situation. Your actions show you are serious.

You cannot control others' behavior, but you can control how you respond to protect your well-being.

6.17 Building Confidence Through Boundaries

Each time you set a boundary or speak assertively, you send a message to yourself that your needs matter. This boosts your self-esteem. Over time, you will notice:

- **Less Resentment**: Because you are not overcommitting or letting people walk all over you.
- **More Energy**: You conserve emotional resources that were once spent pleasing others.
- **Clearer Identity**: You know what you stand for and what you will not tolerate.
- **Better Relationships**: People learn to respect you, and you feel more comfortable sharing your genuine self with them.

Think of boundaries as the glue that holds healthy relationships together. Without them, confusion and resentment can grow.

6.18 Practical Exercises for Assertiveness

1. **Role-Playing**: Ask a trusted friend to practice boundary-setting scenarios with you. For example, have them pretend to be a coworker asking you to work overtime again. Rehearse an assertive response.
2. **Daily "No" Challenge**: Challenge yourself to say "no" to at least one small request that you truly do not want to do. It could be something as simple as refusing an extra chore when you are tired.
3. **Write It Out**: If you struggle to speak up in the moment, try writing a short script. For instance, "I appreciate the offer, but I have to say no because I'm already overbooked."
4. **Observe Others**: Notice friends or colleagues who are good at setting boundaries. What words do they use? How do they handle pushback? Learning from others can make it easier to develop your own style.

CHAPTER 7

Emotional Resilience

7.1 Introduction to Emotional Resilience

Emotional resilience is the ability to recover from stress, setbacks, or hardships. Think of a rubber band that can stretch and return to its original shape. In life, you will face challenges that pull you in different directions. Emotional resilience helps you bounce back when life's pressures become intense.

We all experience losses, failures, or disappointments. Emotional resilience does not mean you never feel sad or upset. Instead, it means that despite difficult feelings, you can eventually find your balance again. Resilient people still cry, feel angry, or worry. But they learn from negative experiences and use those lessons to grow stronger.

Many women juggle multiple roles—caregiver, professional, friend, partner, and more. Emotional resilience can be the glue that holds these roles together, preventing stress in one area of life from overwhelming everything else. By the end of this chapter, you will learn practical ways to build your own resilience, no matter your past experiences or current challenges.

7.2 Why Emotional Resilience Matters for Women

Society often places heavy expectations on women. You might feel pressure to be the perfect parent, an excellent employee, and a supportive friend, all while keeping up with social or cultural traditions. This can lead to constant stress. Emotional resilience is vital because it allows you to handle these pressures without losing your sense of self.

Women also face unique challenges, including bias in the workplace, unequal domestic responsibilities, or cultural norms that discourage openly expressing strong emotions. Some women feel they must "hold it all together" without showing vulnerability. Resilience does not stop you from feeling sad or frustrated; instead, it helps you process those emotions in a healthy way. You can express them, learn from them, and move forward rather than staying stuck.

Additionally, emotional resilience is linked to better mental health. It can help prevent chronic stress or anxiety from turning into more serious problems. By developing resilience, women can protect their emotional well-being, nurture their relationships, and approach life's ups and downs with greater confidence.

7.3 The Mind-Body Connection

Your emotional resilience is closely tied to your physical well-being. When you are stressed, your body might show it through tense muscles, headaches, or an upset stomach. Long-term emotional strain can weaken your immune system and make you more vulnerable to illnesses.

On the other hand, improving your physical health often boosts your resilience. For example, getting regular exercise can release endorphins—often called "feel-good" chemicals—which help you handle stress better. Eating balanced meals can stabilize your mood and energy levels. Even small actions like standing up and stretching during a stressful workday can improve blood flow, reset your mind, and help you regain composure.

This mind-body connection reminds us that building emotional resilience is not just about thoughts or feelings in isolation. It is about treating your whole self with respect. That includes staying hydrated, moving your body, and seeking rest when you are overwhelmed. Each small step you take in caring for your physical side also helps fortify your emotional side.

7.4 The Role of Stress in Testing Resilience

Stress is a normal part of life. Small amounts of stress, like preparing for a job interview or giving a presentation, can even be motivating. But chronic stress—like ongoing financial problems or a toxic work environment—can wear you down over time.

This ongoing tension often tests your resilience. If you handle stress in unhealthy ways—like ignoring it or lashing out at people around you—you may feel more drained and discouraged. But if you use stress as a signal that you need to adjust or seek support, it can become a tool for growth. For instance, if your workload is too heavy, talking to a supervisor about more realistic deadlines can reduce stress and show self-advocacy. That active approach helps strengthen your resilience muscle.

Resilience grows when you see stressful events as opportunities to learn. Ask yourself: "What can this experience teach me?" or "How can I manage this situation in a healthier way?" Over time, each stressor you overcome adds to your pool of confidence. You recognize your own ability to cope, making future stressors less daunting.

7.5 Common Myths About Resilience

1. **Myth**: Resilient people never cry or feel negative emotions.
   Reality: Emotions are normal, and resilient individuals do experience anger, sadness, or worry. The key difference is they do not get stuck in those emotions forever.
2. **Myth**: Resilience is something you are either born with or not.
   Reality: While some people may have an easier time bouncing back, resilience is a skill anyone can build. With practice, you can become more emotionally flexible.
3. **Myth**: Being resilient means you handle everything alone.
   Reality: Seeking help from friends, family, or professionals is often part of resilience. Strong social support can make it easier to face challenges.
4. **Myth**: If you are resilient, you will not be affected by big life events.
   Reality: Major losses or traumas affect everyone. Resilience helps you recover and find hope again, but it does not erase the initial pain.

Recognizing these myths ensures you do not have unrealistic expectations about resilience. You can be resilient and still need to lean on others or take time to grieve.

7.6 Building Emotional Resilience

Building resilience is a gradual process. Below are some strategies:

1. **Develop Healthy Coping Skills**
   Coping skills are the tools you use to handle stress or disappointment. These can include journaling, talking with a trusted friend, practicing relaxation techniques, or working on a hobby. Each time you use a healthy coping strategy instead of avoiding your problems, you strengthen your resilience.
2. **Keep a Balanced Perspective**
   When something bad happens, it can feel like your entire world is crashing down. Try to step back and see the bigger picture. Remind yourself of problems you have solved in the past. This perspective helps you remember that setbacks are often temporary.
3. **Focus on Small Wins**
   Celebrating small victories can build your confidence. Did you manage a tough conversation without losing your cool? Did you finish a project even though you felt like quitting? Recognizing these small achievements shows you that you are more capable than you might believe.
4. **Build and Use Support Systems**
   A strong support system might include family members, friends, mentors, or a community group. Share your challenges with people who genuinely care. When you feel understood and supported, it is easier to keep going.
5. **Practice Self-Compassion**
   Talk to yourself kindly rather than harshly. Acknowledge that you are doing your best under the circumstances. This positive inner voice can help you bounce back more quickly from setbacks.

7.7 The Difference Between Avoidance and Resilience

Sometimes people confuse "not letting things bother you" with true resilience. They might push down their feelings or pretend nothing is wrong. This is **avoidance**, not resilience. Avoidance often leads to bigger problems later. For example, if you never talk about your sadness, it can grow into deeper emotional issues like prolonged depression.

Resilience, on the other hand, involves facing the situation directly. You might feel sad or angry, but you do not hide from those emotions. Instead, you recognize them, work through them (perhaps with help), and then find a path forward. Avoidance is like sweeping dirt under a rug: it might look clean on the surface, but the mess remains underneath. Resilience is more like cleaning the floor properly—you face the dirt, handle it, and truly create a healthier environment.

7.8 Strategies for Handling Emotional Overwhelm

In moments of extreme emotion—when it feels like everything is crashing down—you can take immediate steps to ground yourself:

1. **Pause and Breathe**: *Close your eyes (if possible) and take several deep breaths. Focus on the feeling of air moving in and out. This simple act can help calm your racing mind.*
2. **Label Your Emotion**: *Say to yourself, "I am feeling really angry" or "I am feeling so worried right now." Naming the emotion can make it feel more manageable, as though you have pinned it down for examination.*
3. **Use a Grounding Object**: *Hold a small object like a smooth stone, a soft piece of fabric, or even your keys. Notice its texture, temperature, and weight. This helps shift your attention from a flood of feelings to the present moment.*
4. **Safe Distraction**: *If the emotion feels too overwhelming, do a short activity that engages your mind differently, like a quick puzzle, a few stretches, or writing down five things you see around you.*
5. **Seek Support**: *Reach out to a loved one or a counselor. Even a brief supportive conversation can bring you back to a calmer state.*

These quick strategies are like emotional first aid. They help you regain control so you can address the root issue without being swept away by big feelings.

7.9 The Value of a Growth Mindset in Resilience

A growth mindset is the belief that your abilities and intelligence can improve with effort. This approach can also apply to your emotional life. When you adopt a growth mindset regarding resilience, you tell yourself, "I can learn to handle difficulties better over time."

This mindset shifts how you see mistakes or failures. Instead of viewing them as final judgments on your worth, you see them as stepping stones toward growth. For instance, if you lose a job opportunity, you might think, "This is a chance to learn new skills or refocus my career goals," rather than, "I am not good enough; my life is over."

A growth mindset encourages you to try again after a setback. It invites you to ask, "What can I learn from this?" People with a growth mindset are often more flexible, open to feedback, and willing to adapt—all traits that boost emotional resilience.

7.10 Real-Life Example: Naomi's Story

Naomi was a new mother going through a tough time. Her baby hardly slept at night, and Naomi felt constantly exhausted. On top of that, she worried she was not being a good parent. One evening, she began to cry uncontrollably because she felt so overwhelmed.

Instead of ignoring her feelings, Naomi decided to seek help. She talked to a friend who recommended a local mothers' support group. There, Naomi learned that many new moms experience the same sleepless nights and self-doubt. She also discovered practical tips for helping her baby settle at night and for taking quick naps during the day.

Through this support group, Naomi gained a sense of community. She realized she was not alone, and she found healthy coping skills—like asking her partner for more help and practicing short relaxation exercises when the baby slept. Though parenting remained challenging, Naomi felt stronger and more capable. Her emotional resilience grew because she faced her difficulties head-on and leaned on others for support.

7.11 Creating a Personal Resilience Plan

A personal resilience plan is like a toolkit you can turn to when times get tough. It helps you remember the strategies and support systems you have at your disposal. Here is a simple outline:

1. **Identify Triggers**: Make a list of situations that typically cause you distress (e.g., conflict at work, financial strain, family disagreements).
2. **List Coping Methods**: For each trigger, note healthy ways you can respond. For example, if family arguments often arise, plan to take a five-minute cooling-off break before continuing the conversation.
3. **Gather Resources**: Write down people you can call for help, such as close friends, therapists, or community hotlines. Also include books, websites, or apps that you find calming or informative.
4. **Set Simple Goals**: Add some small but meaningful goals that help you build resilience, like practicing a 10-minute relaxation exercise each day or spending time outdoors once a week.
5. **Check In Regularly**: Look at your plan once a month. See if there are new triggers or better strategies. Adjust as needed.

Having a written or digital resilience plan makes it easier to remember your options when you feel overwhelmed. It is a reassuring reminder that you are not powerless.

7.12 Tools and Tips for Ongoing Practice

1. **Journaling**: Writing regularly about your feelings helps you spot patterns. You might notice that certain times of the year or certain activities cause more stress. Awareness is the first step to handling those triggers better.
2. **Affirmations for Resilience**: Short statements like "I can handle challenges, one step at a time," or "I am learning to adapt and grow," can support a more positive mindset. Repeating them may feel awkward at first, but it can gently reshape your inner dialogue over time.

3. **Mindful Check-Ins**: Once or twice a day, pause and ask, "How am I feeling right now?" If you are tense, take a minute to breathe or stretch. This habit trains you to deal with stress before it becomes overwhelming.
4. **Learn New Skills**: Building skills in problem-solving, communication, or even time management can reduce stress in various parts of your life. Each skill you gain becomes another tool in your resilience toolkit.
5. **Celebrate Progress**: If you handle a tough situation better than you did in the past, acknowledge it. Maybe you overcame an argument with less anger, or you managed a financial hiccup calmly. These successes show that you are capable of growth.

7.13 The Importance of Reflection and Review

Resilience is a journey, not a one-time achievement. Reflecting on your experiences helps you spot progress and areas needing more attention. After handling a crisis or a stressful phase, ask:

- **What did I do well?**
- **Which parts were challenging?**
- **What could I try differently next time?**

This reflection keeps you from repeating the same mistakes. For example, if you realize that procrastination caused you last-minute anxiety, you might commit to a new schedule. Or if you noticed that talking with a specific friend helped you calm down, you can plan to connect with them more often.

7.14 The Impact of Emotional Resilience on Relationships

When you are emotionally resilient, you tend to bring a calmer presence into your relationships. You are more able to listen, empathize, and offer support without being overwhelmed by your own stress. This does not mean you never argue or feel upset, but it does mean you recover from conflicts more quickly and can approach them with a clearer mind.

Resilience also sets an example for people around you. Children, coworkers, or friends might see how you handle tough times and learn from your approach. You become a role model for dealing with life's hurdles in a healthier, more balanced way.

Additionally, resilient people are often better at respecting others' boundaries and emotional needs. Because they practice healthy coping strategies, they typically do not rely on others to "fix" all their problems. This fosters more stable and positive connections, where each person supports the other rather than placing all the burdens on one side.

CHAPTER 8

The Power of Positive Thinking

8.1 What Is Positive Thinking?

Positive thinking is the practice of choosing to look for the good in situations rather than focusing on the bad. It does not mean ignoring problems or pretending that everything is perfect. Instead, it is about directing your energy toward hopeful ideas, solutions, and self-encouragement.

In everyday life, you encounter ups and downs. A positive thinker acknowledges the tough parts but does not let them overshadow the good that may still exist. It is like looking at a partly cloudy sky and noticing the patches of blue. You are not denying the clouds; you are just not ignoring the brighter spots that exist alongside them.

Positive thinking can reshape your experience of daily life. Imagine waking up and saying, "I can handle today's challenges," compared to, "Everything will go wrong." Your mindset influences how you react to the events that follow. By welcoming a more hopeful viewpoint, you often find it easier to cope with stress, spot opportunities, and keep your spirits lifted.

8.2 Why Positive Thinking Matters

The power of positive thinking has several benefits:

1. **Improved Emotional Health**: When you focus on possibility rather than defeat, it is harder for negativity to take root. This can lead to less anxiety, fewer depressive thoughts, and a more steady mood overall.
2. **Better Stress Management**: Positive thinking helps you see problems as challenges you can work on. This shift reduces the feeling of being overwhelmed and keeps you calmer under pressure.
3. **Increased Motivation**: If you believe something is possible, you are more likely to try harder or stick with a task. On the other hand, negative thinking can lead to giving up too soon.

4. **Enhanced Creativity**: A solution-focused mindset naturally leads you to brainstorm new ideas instead of getting stuck in worry. Creativity often thrives when you feel open and optimistic.
5. **Stronger Relationships**: Being around someone who looks for the best in people and situations can be uplifting. Positive thinkers can also better support loved ones by offering hope when difficulties arise.

8.3 Positive Thinking vs. Blind Optimism

It is important to separate **positive thinking** from **blind optimism**. Blind optimism ignores or denies real problems. It might sound like, "Everything will be fine no matter what," without any plan or awareness of the issues at hand. This can lead to a false sense of security and poor decision-making.

Positive thinking recognizes that difficulties exist but chooses a constructive attitude toward handling them. For example, if you have a big project due at work, a positive thinker acknowledges it will be challenging but believes they can figure it out step by step. Blind optimism would say, "I do not need to worry at all. It will magically get done." The difference is subtle but important. Positive thinking still involves action and responsibility.

8.4 The Science of Positive Thoughts

Studies in psychology suggest that people who regularly practice positive thinking are often healthier and happier. This is partly because optimism helps reduce the effects of stress on the body. When you feel hopeful, your body tends to release fewer stress hormones, leading to benefits like lower blood pressure and a healthier immune response.

Positive thoughts can also shape your brain's neural pathways. Over time, if you repeatedly focus on finding solutions and seeing possibilities, your brain becomes better at spotting them quickly. This is sometimes called "neuroplasticity." Essentially, your brain changes based on what you consistently do. So, choosing positive thoughts can, in a real biological sense, help you become more inclined to see potential rather than problems.

8.5 Negative Thinking Patterns

Many people struggle with negative thinking patterns that hinder their progress. Recognizing these patterns is the first step toward change. A few common ones include:

1. **Catastrophizing**: *Imagining the worst possible outcome for any situation. For instance, if you get a minor critique at work, you jump to thinking you will be fired and become homeless.*
2. **Black-and-White Thinking**: *Seeing situations as either all good or all bad. You might think, "If I did not do it perfectly, I have completely failed."*
3. **Overgeneralizing**: *Drawing broad conclusions from one event. If a friend cancels plans, you might decide no one cares about you and that you will never have close relationships.*
4. **Mental Filtering**: *Ignoring positive details and focusing only on the negative. If you receive 10 compliments and 1 criticism, you zero in on the criticism as proof you are terrible.*
5. **Labeling**: *Defining yourself or others using a single negative word, like "I am lazy," or "He is useless," based on one action or shortcoming.*

Identifying these thought patterns allows you to catch them and replace them with more balanced perspectives.

8.6 Shifting from Negative to Positive

Changing negative thoughts into positive ones is a gradual process, but it can be done:

1. **Awareness**: *Notice when you slip into negative thinking. That moment of realization is key.*
2. **Pause and Question**: *Ask yourself if there is real evidence for your negative assumption. Often, negative thoughts exaggerate or ignore key facts.*

3. **Reframe**: Replace the negative statement with a more balanced or hopeful one. For example, swap "I always mess up" for "I sometimes struggle, but I can learn from this."
4. **Practice Regularly**: Write down your negative thoughts and possible positive reframes in a journal. This practice helps train your brain to consider uplifting alternatives.
5. **Celebrate Progress**: Each time you successfully catch and challenge a negative thought, give yourself credit. Small wins add up to big changes over time.

8.7 Daily Habits to Encourage Positive Thinking

1. **Morning Affirmations**: Start the day with a simple, encouraging sentence. It could be, "I am capable of handling whatever comes my way today."
2. **Gratitude Moments**: Pause at least once a day to list a few things you are thankful for—like having a warm bed, a supportive friend, or simply a tasty meal. Focusing on gratitude shifts your attention away from what is lacking.
3. **Positive Environment**: Surround yourself with people, music, and even artwork that inspire you or make you smile. This might mean unfollowing social media accounts that drain your mood and following those that lift you up.
4. **Kind Language**: Pay attention to how you speak about yourself and others. Try to avoid harsh criticism or cynical remarks. Speak with kindness, even if it is just to yourself in private.
5. **Mindful Media Consumption**: Stay informed, but do not overload on negative news. Balance the tough stories with uplifting or educational content.

8.8 Overcoming Obstacles to Positive Thinking

Sometimes, adopting a more optimistic view can be challenging:

- **Long-Standing Negative Beliefs**: *If you grew up in an environment where criticism and worry were the norms, it might feel unnatural to focus on the positive.*
- **Chronic Stress**: *Persistent problems—like financial struggles or health issues—can overshadow any optimism.*
- **Mental Health Conditions**: *Conditions like depression or anxiety can make it harder to maintain hope.*

In such cases, you might need extra support from counselors, self-help groups, or mental health professionals. Positive thinking does not replace professional care, but it can be a valuable complement to therapy or medication if needed. By combining professional help with your own effort to shift thoughts, you can make steady progress.

8.9 Real-Life Example: Aria's Turnaround

Aria was an art student who constantly worried she was not good enough. She compared her work to everyone else's and believed she lacked talent. Over time, these negative thoughts paralyzed her creativity. She avoided trying new art techniques, fearing failure.

One of Aria's teachers noticed her frustration and suggested she keep a "success sketchbook." In this sketchbook, Aria drew or wrote down one art-related success each day—no matter how small. Some days, she noted, "I learned a new shading method," or "A classmate liked my painting." At first, Aria felt silly doing it. But after a few weeks, she noticed her achievements were piling up.

This daily habit fed her confidence. When negative thoughts like "I cannot draw hands well" appeared, she would remind herself of the day she drew a hand and received a compliment from a friend. Slowly, her mindset shifted from fear to curiosity. She started experimenting with styles she used to avoid. Aria still had moments of doubt, but her overall outlook became much brighter. She discovered that by directing her focus toward her progress and possibilities, she could push through the fear of failing.

8.10 Long-Term Benefits of Positive Thinking

Thinking positively on a regular basis can bring many long-term advantages:

1. **Higher Resilience**: As you maintain an optimistic viewpoint, you tend to bounce back from problems more easily.
2. **Better Physical Health**: Lower stress can translate to fewer tension headaches, better sleep, and a stronger immune system.
3. **Enhanced Creativity and Productivity**: A hopeful outlook makes it easier to brainstorm ideas and stay motivated on tasks.
4. **Stronger Social Connections**: People are often drawn to those who can see the bright side, making it easier to form and maintain fulfilling relationships.
5. **Greater Overall Life Satisfaction**: Over time, focusing on the positive can lead to a more content and joyful life, even during stressful periods.

8.11 Combining Positive Thinking with Realistic Action

Positive thinking should go hand in hand with action. Simply believing something will get better without taking steps to improve it can lead to disappointment. For example, if you want a new job, positive thinking might help you say, "I can learn the skills needed." But you also need to apply for positions, update your resume, and prepare for interviews.

When combined, optimism and action create a powerful force. Optimism fuels the energy to act, and action validates that optimism by leading to real-world results. This teamwork between mind and effort can help you move forward even in challenging situations.

8.12 Common Pitfalls When Trying to Think Positively

1. **Ignoring Genuine Problems**: Refusing to see an actual problem will not make it go away. Acknowledge the issue, then approach it with a solutions-focused mindset.

2. **Downplaying Others' Feelings**: Sometimes, a well-meaning positive thinker might dismiss a friend's worries by saying, "You just need to be more positive." This can make them feel unheard. Listening and empathy should come before offering optimistic advice.
3. **Expecting Instant Results**: Switching from negative thinking to positive thinking is a journey. You may not see big changes in your outlook overnight, but small steps do add up.
4. **Comparing Your Journey**: Each person's path to positivity is unique. If you see someone else succeed faster, do not assume you are failing. Keep focusing on your own growth.

8.13 Ways to Sustain a Positive Outlook

1. **Review Your Goals**: Regularly check your personal goals to remind yourself of what you are working toward. This keeps your mind focused on possibilities.
2. **Stay Curious**: Ask questions like, "What if this turns out better than I expected?" or "How else can I look at this situation?" Curiosity breaks negative loops.
3. **Reflect on Growth**: Whenever you handle a tough situation better than before, note it. Maybe you stayed calm during an argument or found a creative workaround for a sudden problem. Recognize these wins.
4. **Foster Supportive Relationships**: Maintain ties with people who encourage your positive mindset. This does not mean you only surround yourself with "yes-people," but rather those who are constructive, not constantly pessimistic.
5. **Learn from Setbacks**: After something goes wrong, instead of dwelling on your mistakes, ask what you can take away to do better next time. Positive thinking sees failure as feedback, not the end.

8.14 A Simple Exercise to Shift Your Mindset

Try this short daily practice:

1. **Name a Challenge**: Think about a problem or worry you currently have.

2. **List the Negative Thoughts**: On a piece of paper, write down all the worries or negative ideas you have about it, like "I might fail," or "People will judge me."
3. **Find a Counterbalance**: Next to each negative point, write a realistic but positive counter-thought. For instance, change "I might fail" to "I can prepare well and learn as I go."
4. **Reflect**: Notice how seeing both the negative thought and its counterbalance side by side feels. You will likely experience a sense of relief or possibility.
5. **Take One Action**: To reinforce this positive mindset, do a small action that moves you forward on the challenge—like making a phone call, sending an email, or doing five minutes of research.

Repeat this process whenever you feel stuck in negativity. Over time, it trains you to look for balanced, hopeful perspectives instead of letting negative ones rule your mind.

8.15 Balancing Hope and Realism

Remember that positive thinking is about balance. You do not want to ignore risks or disregard reality. Instead, you want to remain open to the best possible outcome while preparing for potential bumps in the road. This balanced approach might look like:

- **Hopeful Thought**: "I can run a half-marathon if I train properly."
- **Realistic Action**: Planning a running schedule, staying hydrated, and gradually increasing distance.

This blend of hope and realism keeps you motivated and mindful at the same time. You do not become naive or overconfident; you simply allow room for success and growth in your plan.

8.16 How Positive Thinking Affects Relationships

A positive mindset can greatly impact how you interact with loved ones and coworkers:

1. **Less Conflict**: You are more likely to approach disagreements calmly, looking for solutions instead of assigning blame.
2. **Better Communication**: Optimism makes it easier to express gratitude, apologize when needed, and show genuine support.
3. **Stronger Empathy**: When you are not bogged down by negativity, you have more emotional energy to understand others and be there for them.
4. **Increased Joy**: Sharing even small joys—like a funny moment or a minor achievement—becomes a way to bond. Positive energy often spreads, lifting the mood of those around you.

As you shift your thinking, you might notice people respond more warmly. They may appreciate your balanced optimism and find it easier to confide in you. This does not mean you must always be cheerful, but consistently practicing positivity can foster deeper and more supportive connections.

8.17 External Reminders and Tools

You can use various tools to keep your mindset positive:

- **Vision Board**: Collect images, words, and quotes that represent your goals and hopes. Put them on a board in a spot you see daily.
- **Phone Alerts**: Set calendar reminders with uplifting phrases. When the alert pops up, pause and reflect on it.
- **App Journals**: Some apps guide you through daily gratitude lists, positive affirmations, or short reflections.
- **Inspirational Reading**: Keep a favorite motivational book or set of quotes handy. Skimming through a few pages can shift your mood when you are feeling negative.

These external supports are like signposts that help you stay on track when your mind starts drifting into doubt or worry.

8.18 Can You Be Too Positive?

In rare cases, people worry about being "too positive." This might happen if positivity leads them to ignore real problems or avoid necessary conflict. For instance, if a close friend constantly disrespects you, responding with forced cheer instead of honest communication could worsen the relationship.

Real positivity recognizes when change is needed and addresses issues openly. It keeps hope alive but does not turn a blind eye to what must be fixed. So, if you find yourself using positivity as an excuse to avoid confronting important problems, it is time to step back and adjust.

8.19 Celebrating Your Positive Shifts

Whenever you notice a positive shift in your thinking—like calming yourself during a tough meeting, focusing on a solution instead of a complaint, or showing kindness to yourself after a mistake—celebrate it. Give yourself a silent cheer or treat yourself to something small you enjoy. These moments reinforce the new pattern in your brain.

Celebration does not have to be big. It could be a quiet acknowledgment: "I handled that well." Over time, these tiny "wins" remind you that progress is happening, and that positivity is a habit you can strengthen.

CHAPTER 9

Strengthening Your Communication Skills

9.1 Introduction to Communication Skills

Communication is how we share thoughts, feelings, and ideas with others. It can be through words, body language, or even facial expressions. Strong communication skills help you express yourself clearly, reduce misunderstandings, and build healthy relationships in every area of life—work, family, friends, and more. But many women struggle to find the right words or speak up when needed. This chapter will explore practical ways you can improve how you communicate, so you feel more confident and understood.

Communication is not just about speaking; it is also about listening, observing, and understanding context. Sometimes the most powerful communicators are not the loudest but those who can clearly express their message while also hearing what others say. By the end of this chapter, you will have tools and insights to enhance your voice, become a better listener, and navigate difficult conversations more effectively.

9.2 Why Communication Matters for Confidence

Communication and confidence go hand in hand. When you can speak up in a clear, concise way, you feel more self-assured. Others also respond better because they see you as someone who knows her mind and respects herself. On the other side, if you struggle to get your message across, you might feel misunderstood or overlooked. That can lower your self-esteem over time.

A confident communicator can say "no" when necessary and "yes" when it feels right, without guilt or confusion. She can give constructive feedback at work, handle disagreements with friends, or discuss important issues with family members. Each time you effectively communicate, you show yourself—and those around you—that your voice matters. This validation can boost your confidence even further, creating a positive cycle of self-belief and strong connections.

9.3 The Basics of Effective Communication

Being an effective communicator involves several basic skills:

1. **Clarity**: Use simple words and a clear structure. Avoid rambling. If you catch yourself talking in circles, pause, gather your thoughts, and begin again.
2. **Listening Actively**: True communication is a two-way street. Show genuine interest in the other person's words by making eye contact, nodding, or offering short verbal acknowledgments like "I see" or "I understand."
3. **Respect**: Even if you disagree, address the other person's perspective calmly. A respectful tone creates an environment where it's safe for both parties to share and explore ideas.
4. **Empathy**: Try to put yourself in the other person's shoes. How do they feel? What do they need from you in that moment? Empathy helps you respond in a way that acknowledges their concerns.
5. **Feedback**: Check to see if you have been understood. You might say, "Let me know if I'm being clear," or, "Does this make sense to you?" This encourages the other person to ask questions if needed.

When these core elements come together, you create a conversation that feels balanced, clear, and productive.

9.4 Overcoming Common Communication Barriers

Communication barriers are things that keep you from sharing or understanding messages effectively. Here are a few and how you can overcome them:

1. **Fear of Judgment**
    - **Barrier**: You worry about what others think, so you stay quiet or water down your message.

- **Solution**: Remind yourself that everyone has a right to express themselves. Start small—speak up in low-pressure settings, like a friendly discussion among close friends. Gradually move to bigger conversations.
2. **Unclear Language**
    - **Barrier**: Overusing jargon, vague terms, or filler words can confuse your listener.
    - **Solution**: Keep it simple. Know your main point before you start talking. Use examples or stories to clarify complex ideas.
3. **Assumptions**
    - **Barrier**: You assume you know what the other person feels or thinks without actually asking.
    - **Solution**: Ask open-ended questions like, "How do you see this issue?" or "Can you tell me more about your point of view?" This invites them to share rather than letting you guess.
4. **Emotional Reactions**
    - **Barrier**: Strong emotions, like anger or frustration, can cause you to shut down or explode.
    - **Solution**: Pause before you speak. Take a deep breath or politely ask for a moment if you need to calm down. Return to the discussion when you are more composed.

By actively addressing these barriers, you open the door to smoother, more fruitful interactions.

9.5 Listening: The Unsung Hero of Good Communication

Many people focus on speaking well but forget that listening is equally critical. Good listening goes beyond just hearing words; it involves understanding feelings, motivations, and context. Here are some strategies:

1. **Active Listening**: Show you are engaged. Maintain eye contact, nod, or say brief confirmations like "Yes," "I see," or "That makes sense." This tells the speaker you are present.
2. **No Interruptions**: Let the other person finish their thought before you jump in. Interrupting signals impatience or disrespect.
3. **Clarifying Questions**: If something is unclear, ask politely: "When you say X, do you mean...?" This prevents misunderstandings.

4. **Reflect Back**: Sometimes called "mirroring," this technique involves repeating what the speaker said in your own words. "So you feel upset because your ideas weren't considered, right?" This validates their feelings.
5. **Stay Open-Minded**: Even if you disagree, try to understand why the other person holds their view. You might learn something new or find common ground.

Strong listening skills can improve your relationships significantly. People appreciate being heard and understood, which often increases the respect they have for you.

9.6 Assertive Communication Techniques

Assertiveness is when you express your thoughts and needs honestly while respecting others. Below are a few specific methods:

1. **"I" Statements**
   Instead of pointing fingers with "You did this" or "You made me feel that," phrase your concerns using "I." For example, "I feel upset when you don't tell me you'll be late, because I worry something happened." This approach focuses on your feelings rather than blaming the other person.
2. **Calm Tone and Body Language**
   Your words matter, but so does how you say them. Keep your posture upright, make gentle eye contact, and speak in a firm but calm voice. Crossing your arms or rolling your eyes sends a contradictory message.
3. **Clear Boundaries**
   If you need to set a limit, be direct: "I'm not comfortable discussing this anymore," or "I can't meet you today because I have other commitments." Offer alternatives if you want, but don't feel pressured to justify yourself endlessly.
4. **Focus on Solutions**
   Assertive communication aims to move toward a mutually agreeable outcome. If you have a complaint, suggest a remedy. For instance, "It would help me if we could plan at least a day in advance."

5. **Reiterate Respect**
   You can be assertive without being rude. A simple statement like, "I respect your feelings, and I also need you to respect mine," can go a long way in keeping the conversation balanced.

Mastering assertive communication can boost your confidence and help you maintain healthier relationships.

9.7 Communicating in Challenging Situations

Not all conversations are easy. Some are highly emotional—discussing conflicts, delivering bad news, or handling sensitive topics. Here's how to navigate those:

1. **Choose the Right Time and Place**
   If possible, pick a private or neutral area where both parties feel safe. Avoid trying to resolve a serious argument in a crowded restaurant or when you are both rushing.
2. **Stay on Topic**
   Keep the conversation focused on the current issue. Bringing up old grudges or unrelated complaints can complicate things and lead to more tension.
3. **Acknowledge Emotions**
   If the other person is upset, a gentle acknowledgment, like "I can see you're really hurt by this," can calm the situation. It shows you care about their emotional state.
4. **Suggest Next Steps**
   Do not end the conversation with unsolved tension. Ask, "What can we do to move forward?" or "How can we prevent this issue in the future?" This turns a difficult moment into a problem-solving session.
5. **Know When to Take a Break**
   If tempers flare, it might help to pause. Suggest continuing the discussion after you both have cooled down or had time to reflect.

Challenging conversations do not have to end in anger or tears. With a calm approach and a willingness to listen, you can turn them into opportunities for growth and understanding.

9.8 Nonverbal Communication: The Unspoken Messages

Words are only one piece of the communication puzzle. Your body language, facial expressions, and even your tone of voice all convey information. Here are some nonverbal cues to be aware of:

1. **Posture**
   Standing or sitting up straight shows confidence. Slouching or crossing your arms can appear defensive or disengaged. If you want to seem approachable, try a more open posture with arms at your sides or gently folded on your lap.
2. **Facial Expressions**
   Smiling can create a friendly atmosphere, but it should match the context. Raising your eyebrows might indicate surprise or doubt. Pay attention to how your face might be sending signals you do not intend.
3. **Eye Contact**
   Looking someone in the eye generally conveys honesty and attentiveness. But remember to balance it—staring too intensely can feel aggressive, while avoiding eye contact might seem like you are hiding something.
4. **Gestures**
   Hand movements can emphasize your points but overdoing it can distract from your message. Keep gestures natural and purposeful.
5. **Tone and Volume**
   A calm, moderate tone often works best. Speaking too quietly suggests uncertainty, while shouting can be intimidating. Aim for a steady voice that people can easily follow.

Being mindful of your nonverbal cues can add power to your words and strengthen how others perceive you.

9.9 Communication in Different Settings

We communicate in many places: at work, with friends, during a conflict, or even on social media. Adapting your style to fit the setting can improve your effectiveness:

1. **Workplace**
     - **Formal Tone**: In professional settings, using clear, structured language is important. Avoid too much slang.
     - **Email Etiquette**: Keep messages concise. Use proper greetings and sign-offs. Proofread for clarity.
     - **Meetings**: Speak up at least once if you have ideas or relevant feedback. This helps you stay visible and engaged.
2. **Family and Close Friends**
     - **Casual Tone**: It's okay to be more relaxed, but remain respectful.
     - **Honesty**: Loved ones often value sincerity. If something bothers you, address it kindly but directly rather than bottling it up.
     - **Quality Listening**: Because emotions can run high in families, good listening prevents misunderstandings.
3. **Social Media and Online**
     - **Clarity in Text**: Tone can be misunderstood in written messages. Use simple language and polite phrasing.
     - **Respect Boundaries**: Not everyone wants personal discussions in public posts. Consider using private messaging for deeper topics.
     - **Pause Before Posting**: Online conflicts can escalate quickly. Think carefully before you respond to avoid heated back-and-forth that solves nothing.

Adjusting your communication style does not mean being fake. It is simply acknowledging that each context has its own expectations and challenges.

9.10 Tips for Improving Public Speaking

Speaking in front of a group—whether it's 5 or 50 people—can be daunting. However, effective public speaking can boost your confidence and open doors. Here are some pointers:

1. **Preparation**
     - **Know Your Topic**: Research and organize your points. Confidence grows when you are well-informed.
     - **Practice Out Loud**: Rehearse your speech or presentation. Record yourself if possible to identify unclear sections.

2. **Structure**
   - **Clear Beginning**: Open with a short overview or an attention-grabbing statement.
   - **Middle Points**: Present your main ideas in a logical order. Use examples to keep the audience engaged.
   - **Conclusion**: Summarize key points and give a memorable final thought or call to action.
3. **Delivery**
   - **Steady Pace**: Avoid speaking too fast, which can happen when you are nervous. A relaxed pace helps listeners follow along.
   - **Eye Contact**: Shift your gaze around the audience. Focusing only on your notes can seem unwelcoming.
   - **Natural Gestures**: Move your hands or walk a bit if it helps you relax, but do not overdo it. Keep your movements purposeful.
4. **Dealing with Nerves**
   - **Practice Breathing Techniques**: A few deep breaths before you start can calm jitters.
   - **Positive Visualization**: Imagine yourself speaking clearly and confidently. This mental rehearsal can ease anxiety.
   - **Focus on Helping**: Think about the value you are providing to the audience, rather than worrying about how you look or sound.

Public speaking is a learnable skill. Over time, these methods can make you more comfortable and allow your message to shine.

9.11 Handling Criticism and Difficult Feedback

No matter how well you speak or listen, there will be times when people criticize you or give feedback you may not want to hear. Here is how to handle it gracefully:

1. **Stay Calm**
   If you feel attacked, you may get defensive. Pause, breathe, and remember that feedback can sometimes lead to improvement.
2. **Listen Fully**
   Do not cut the person off. Let them finish explaining. They might have a perspective you have never considered.

3. **Ask Clarifying Questions**
   If the feedback is vague—"You're not doing well"—ask for specifics: "Could you give me an example of what I can improve?"
4. **Thank Them**
   Even if you disagree, acknowledging the effort they took to share their viewpoint can cool down tension. You can say, "I appreciate you telling me this."
5. **Decide What to Take Onboard**
   Not all criticism is useful. Some might be based on personal bias or unrealistic expectations. Consider the source and content carefully. If you think it can help you, adapt. If not, let it go.

Learning to respond well to criticism shows maturity and keeps communication lines open.

9.12 Balancing Talking and Listening

Sometimes, people mistake good communication for being the one who talks the most. In reality, strong communicators know how to balance speaking and listening:

1. **Be Aware of Your Share**
   Pay attention to how long you speak in group settings. If you dominate the conversation, others might feel shut out. If you never speak, you miss chances to contribute.
2. **Ask for Input**
   If you notice someone is quiet, you can gently invite them in: "Sarah, do you have thoughts on this?" This not only balances conversation but also shows respect.
3. **Practice Self-Checking**
   Are you listening attentively, or waiting to talk again? Pause and let others finish. If a thought pops into your head, hold it for a second instead of interrupting.
4. **Quality Over Quantity**
   It's not about how many words you say, but the value of those words. A few well-chosen sentences can be more powerful than a long, rambling speech.

Maintaining this give-and-take rhythm fosters mutual respect and more satisfying discussions.

9.13 Cultural and Individual Differences

Everyone you communicate with has a different background, personality, and outlook. Being sensitive to these differences can boost your effectiveness:

1. **Cultural Norms**
   Some cultures encourage direct, straightforward talk, while others value subtlety and "saving face." If you are speaking with someone from a different background, be observant. Ask polite questions about their preferences if needed.
2. **Personality Variances**
   Introverts may need more time to process thoughts before speaking. Extroverts might think aloud. Adapting your pace can help everyone feel comfortable.
3. **Language Barriers**
   When someone is speaking a second language, or you are, slow down, choose simpler words, and be patient. Check that both sides understand.
4. **Conflict Styles**
   Some individuals prefer immediate confrontation to resolve issues, while others avoid direct conflict. Learning these styles can help you approach disagreements more productively.

Remember, no one approach suits every person. Flexibility is key to inclusive and respectful communication.

9.14 Building Trust Through Communication

Trust is the bedrock of strong relationships, both personal and professional. Communication plays a huge role in forming and maintaining that trust:

1. **Consistency**
   If you say you will do something, follow through. Broken promises damage credibility faster than almost anything else.
2. **Transparency**
   Share information openly when you can. Hiding details or giving half-truths can make people suspect you have something to conceal.
3. **Confidentiality**
   If someone shares something private, respect their privacy. Gossiping or revealing secrets erodes trust.
4. **Positive Acknowledgment**
   Recognize others' efforts or achievements. This genuine praise shows you see and value their contributions, deepening mutual respect.

When people trust you, they are more open to what you have to say and more likely to share honestly in return.

9.15 Practice Exercises for Better Communication

1. **Record Yourself**
   Use your phone to record a short speech or even a conversation role-play. Listen afterward. Note if you used filler words like "um" or "like" excessively, or if your tone sounded overly hesitant.
2. **Journal Your Experiences**
   After a meaningful conversation (good or bad), jot down what went well and what could improve. This reflection helps you see patterns in your interactions.
3. **Try "Mirroring" in Real-Time**
   In a friendly chat, practice restating what the other person says in your own words before responding. This hones your listening and helps them feel heard.
4. **Set Specific Goals**
   Maybe you want to speak up at least once in each work meeting or share an idea with a friend group. Create small, achievable aims for each day or week.
5. **Attend Workshops or Clubs**
   If public speaking is a goal, groups like Toastmasters or local workshops on communication can offer structured practice and feedback.

Regular, conscious practice can transform your communication style over time.

9.16 Real-Life Example: Danielle's Growth

Danielle worked in an office where her boss often overlooked her ideas. She felt frustrated but rarely spoke up. Finally, she decided to improve her communication. She started by noting down her ideas before meetings and giving herself a personal rule: she had to share at least one idea each time. When she did, she used an assertive but calm tone, stating, "I believe this approach could save time" or "I have a different view to consider."

At first, her boss seemed surprised. However, Danielle kept at it. She listened actively to her boss's feedback, acknowledging valid points but standing firm when she felt confident in her perspective. Over a few months, her colleagues began to notice her contributions. Her boss started asking for her input directly. Danielle's self-esteem rose as she became a recognized voice in the office. What changed? She used her voice and listened thoughtfully, turning a challenging environment into a space where her input mattered.

9.17 Measuring Your Communication Progress

It can be helpful to track your growth:

- **Reduced Misunderstandings**: Are people asking fewer questions to clarify your words? This could mean you are getting clearer.
- **More Engagement**: Do people respond more positively or ask for your opinion more often? This may mean your confidence and clarity are shining through.
- **Feedback**: Ask trusted friends or colleagues for honest feedback: "How do you think I'm doing with speaking up or listening?"
- **Personal Feelings**: Notice if you feel calmer and more in control during conversations. Emotional ease often signals improved communication.

Celebrating these improvements boosts motivation to keep refining your skills.

9.18 Communication's Impact on Confidence and Relationships

As you strengthen your communication, you will likely notice:

1. **Greater Self-Respect**: Expressing your thoughts and needs affirms your sense of worth. You recognize that you deserve to be heard.
2. **Improved Teamwork**: Whether at work or in personal partnerships, clear communication fosters collaboration and reduces friction.
3. **Deeper Connections**: When people see you genuinely listen and share respectfully, they feel safer opening up. Relationships become richer.
4. **Less Regret**: Instead of leaving conversations feeling, "I should have said something," you will know you spoke your truth in a respectful way.
5. **Boosted Morale**: Good communication often leads to positive outcomes—less conflict, more solutions, and a smoother flow of ideas.

Over time, these benefits ripple out, uplifting other areas of your life as well.

9.19 Overcoming Setbacks

Even with the best intentions, communication can still go wrong:

- **Heated Arguments**: Sometimes discussions become emotional. If you slip into yelling or crying, you can still salvage the conversation. Apologize if needed, take a break, and try again later.
- **Misinterpretations**: You might say something you consider harmless, but the other person hears an insult. Slow down, clarify, and apologize if you caused offense.
- **Progress Takes Time**: Do not be discouraged if you do not become a master communicator overnight. It is a journey. Each small step matters.

The key is to learn from mistakes and keep practicing. Over time, you will see improvement in how smoothly you handle various talks.

CHAPTER 10

Managing Fear and Stress

10.1 Understanding Fear and Stress

Fear and stress are natural parts of life. Fear is usually triggered by a perceived threat or danger—real or imagined—while stress often arises from pressure or demands placed upon you. Both can serve useful purposes: fear can keep you safe from potential harm, and stress can motivate you to meet deadlines or solve problems. However, when these feelings become overwhelming or persistent, they can harm your health, relationships, and overall happiness.

Many women find themselves juggling roles and expectations, which can amplify feelings of stress. You might worry about finances, family obligations, job performance, or personal safety. Over time, too much fear or stress can lead to physical problems like headaches, insomnia, and weakened immunity, as well as emotional challenges such as anxiety and burnout. This chapter explores practical ways to manage fear and stress so you can enjoy a calmer, more fulfilling life.

10.2 Why It's Important to Tackle Fear and Stress

1. **Better Health**: Chronic stress increases the risk of serious health issues, including heart disease, high blood pressure, and depression. Handling stress can boost your immune system and energy levels.
2. **Stronger Relationships**: When fear or stress is high, patience often runs low. You might snap at loved ones or shut down emotionally. Learning to cope can improve communication and connection.
3. **Enhanced Productivity**: Stress can sap your concentration and creativity. Reducing it frees up mental space, allowing you to be more effective at work or in personal projects.
4. **Greater Confidence**: Constant fear undermines your belief in yourself. Overcoming these worries helps you trust your abilities and decisions, fueling growth in every area of life.

5. **Emotional Balance**: *Managing stress allows you to experience life's highs and lows more smoothly, rather than swinging between extremes of anxiety and exhaustion.*

Addressing fear and stress is a key step in leading a balanced, empowered life. By learning to manage these forces, you give yourself the freedom to explore, take healthy risks, and grow.

10.3 Common Causes of Fear and Stress

1. **Financial Pressure**: Concerns about paying bills, saving for the future, or managing debt can be significant sources of stress.
2. **Work or Career Issues**: Tight deadlines, heavy workloads, or conflicts with colleagues can create ongoing tension.
3. **Family Responsibilities**: Caring for children, elderly parents, or handling household tasks can become overwhelming, especially when combined with other duties.
4. **Health Problems**: Chronic illness, acute medical conditions, or fear of becoming sick can lead to ongoing worry.
5. **Uncertainty or Change**: Moving to a new city, starting a different job, or going through relationship changes can trigger anxiety.

Recognizing where your fear or stress comes from can be a powerful first step. Once you identify the source, you can focus on strategies that directly address your situation.

10.4 Physical and Emotional Signs of Stress Overload

It is easy to ignore stress until it becomes unmanageable. Knowing the warning signs can help you act sooner:

- **Physical Signs**: Headaches, upset stomach, tense muscles, back pain, frequent colds or illnesses, changes in appetite or sleep.
- **Emotional Signs**: Feeling irritable or moody, crying unexpectedly, becoming overly sensitive to criticism, or losing interest in activities you once enjoyed.

- **Mental Signs**: Racing thoughts, difficulty concentrating, forgetfulness, persistent negative self-talk.
- **Behavioral Signs**: Withdrawing from social events, using alcohol or other substances to cope, procrastinating important tasks.

If you notice these signs regularly, it is a signal that your stress level is too high. The good news is you can intervene with healthy coping methods before matters get worse.

10.5 Healthy Coping Techniques

Managing fear and stress involves discovering methods that relax the body and calm the mind. Some popular, research-backed approaches include:

1. **Deep Breathing Exercises**
    - **How It Works**: Slow, deep breaths can signal your body to relax. When stressed, people often take quick, shallow breaths, which can make anxiety worse.
    - **Try It**: Inhale for a count of 4, hold for 2, then exhale for a count of 4. Repeat for a minute or more.
2. **Progressive Muscle Relaxation (PMR)**
    - **How It Works**: You systematically tense and then release each muscle group, from your toes up to your head. This releases physical tension that often comes with stress.
    - **Try It**: Sit or lie down, tense your feet for 5 seconds, then let go. Move to calves, thighs, and so on. Pay attention to the difference between tension and relaxation.
3. **Mindful Meditation**
    - **How It Works**: By focusing on the present moment—your breath, a repeated word (mantra), or the environment—you quiet the racing thoughts that fuel stress.
    - **Try It**: Sit comfortably, close your eyes, and focus on your inhale and exhale. If your mind drifts, gently bring it back to your breath.
4. **Guided Imagery**
    - **How It Works**: You imagine a peaceful scene in vivid detail. This mental escape can counteract stressful thoughts.

        ○ **Try It**: Picture a calm beach or a cozy cabin in the woods. Engage all your senses—what do you see, hear, smell, and feel?
   5. **Physical Activities**
        ○ **How It Works**: Exercise releases endorphins, helps burn off nervous energy, and can clear the mind.
        ○ **Try It**: Choose an activity you enjoy—dancing, walking, swimming, or yoga. Even a short 10-minute walk can reduce stress.

Experiment with these techniques to find which combination works best for you. You might prefer quick breathing exercises when anxious at work, while PMR might help you unwind before bed.

10.6 Creating a Support System

A strong support network can help you navigate fearful or stressful times more effectively. This may include:

- **Friends and Family**: People who genuinely care about you can offer a listening ear or practical help, like babysitting while you run errands.
- **Support Groups**: Local or online communities can connect you with those who have faced similar issues. Sharing stories and coping tips can be comforting.
- **Professional Help**: Therapists, counselors, or coaches can provide guidance tailored to your specific needs. They have training in stress management techniques and can offer insights you might not see on your own.
- **Spiritual or Community Resources**: Religious leaders, community centers, or volunteer groups can also be sources of emotional support or advice.

Reaching out for help is not a sign of weakness. It shows courage and wisdom to know when you need an extra hand.

10.7 Challenging Negative Thoughts That Drive Fear

Sometimes fear stems not from actual danger but from negative or exaggerated thoughts. Learning to question these thoughts can reduce worry:

1. **Identify the Thought**: Write it down—"I'll fail this test," "I'll never find a better job," or "People will judge me."
2. **Ask for Evidence**: Is there real proof this will happen? Could there be a different outcome?
3. **Consider Alternatives**: Maybe you will pass the test if you study, or maybe some people will judge you, but many will not.
4. **Reframe**: Turn "I'm definitely going to fail" into "I have a chance to succeed if I prepare and ask for help."

Over time, consistently reframing negative thoughts teaches your mind to see possibilities instead of assuming the worst.

10.8 Time Management to Reduce Stress

Poor time management is a common cause of stress. When tasks pile up, anxiety often follows. Here are tips to stay organized:

1. **Prioritize Tasks**
   Make a list of what you must do, ordered by importance or deadline. Focus on the top items first.
2. **Break Large Projects Down**
   Big tasks can feel overwhelming. Divide them into smaller steps, and celebrate each mini-completion.
3. **Use a Planner or App**
   Writing tasks in a calendar or using a digital tool can give you a clear view of what lies ahead. It also prevents you from forgetting important dates.
4. **Set Realistic Goals**
   Do not try to do everything at once. Overloading yourself is a recipe for failure and more stress.
5. **Allocate Buffer Time**
   Life rarely goes exactly as planned. Include small breaks or extra time between tasks to handle surprises without panic.

Learning to manage your schedule effectively can free you from constant last-minute rushing, giving you more mental and emotional space.

10.9 Practical Strategies to Face Fear

Some fears hold you back, such as fear of public speaking, fear of rejection, or fear of change. These strategies can help you face them:

1. **Gradual Exposure**
   Ease into what scares you in small, controlled steps. If you fear public speaking, start by giving a short talk to a friend, then move to a small group, and so on.
2. **Positive Role Models**
   Observe someone who handles the feared activity well. Learn from their approach, or even ask for tips.
3. **Rewrite the Story**
   Tell yourself a different narrative: "I'm capable of learning this skill," rather than "I'm doomed to fail." Visualize success.
4. **Set a Challenge**
   Treat the fear like a personal challenge. "I want to push myself to see what I'm really capable of." This reframes fear as an opportunity for growth.
5. **Reward Yourself**
   Celebrate each step you take toward conquering your fear, whether that's trying a new activity or speaking up in a meeting. A small treat or personal acknowledgment can reinforce your bravery.

Facing fear is rarely easy, but each victory builds confidence and teaches you that you are stronger than you might think.

10.10 Lifestyle Habits That Support Stress Management

Your daily habits can either increase or decrease stress. Consider adding these supportive routines:

1. **Quality Sleep**
   Aim for 7-9 hours a night. Lack of sleep can weaken your resilience, making you more sensitive to stress.
2. **Balanced Diet**
   Eating a variety of fruits, vegetables, whole grains, and protein can stabilize your energy and mood. High-sugar or high-caffeine diets may worsen stress symptoms.
3. **Regular Exercise**
   Even moderate physical activity—like walking or yoga—can reduce tension, clear your mind, and boost your mood.
4. **Limit Stimulants**
   Too much caffeine or nicotine can increase heart rate and make anxiety symptoms stronger.
5. **Set Boundaries**
   Give yourself downtime. Constantly checking work emails or trying to do everything for everyone else is exhausting. Protect your personal space and leisure time.

A healthy lifestyle forms a strong foundation, making it easier to cope with stress whenever it arises.

10.11 The Power of Relaxation and Downtime

In a busy world, downtime can feel like a luxury, but it's actually essential:

1. **Relaxation Techniques**
   Activities like reading, listening to music, drawing, or taking a warm bath can calm your nervous system. These moments act as a pressure valve for built-up stress.
2. **Mindful Breaks**
   Rather than scrolling your phone during breaks, try a brief mindfulness session—focus on your surroundings, breathe slowly, and let any racing thoughts pass by without dwelling on them.
3. **Short Vacations or Staycations**
   If possible, take a day off now and then to recharge. Even a "staycation" at home, where you avoid chores and just relax, can significantly reduce stress.

4. **Scheduled Fun**
   Treat enjoyable activities like important appointments. Whether it's a hobby, a meet-up with friends, or a family game night, schedule it so you do not keep putting it off.

By regularly refilling your emotional and mental tank, you're better prepared to handle everyday stressors.

10.12 Handling Sudden Anxiety or Panic

Sometimes fear or stress hits like a wave—sudden and intense. Quick tools to regain control include:

1. **Focus on One Object**
   Choose something nearby—a pen, a cup, a painting—and study it closely. Notice every detail, color, or texture. This grounding technique reduces swirling thoughts.
2. **Count Backwards**
   Slowly count from 10 down to 1. Imagine each number dissolving in your mind as you exhale. This can slow a racing heartbeat.
3. **Name Three Things**
   Name three things you see, three things you hear, and three things you can touch. This returns your awareness to the present moment.
4. **Affirmations**
   Repeat short phrases like, "I am safe right now," or "This feeling will pass." Speak them in your mind or out loud if you're alone.
5. **Seek Help If Needed**
   If panic attacks or extreme anxiety happen often, consult a mental health professional. They can guide you through therapies like cognitive-behavioral therapy (CBT) or medication if necessary.

These quick methods can help you ride out moments of acute fear until your mind and body settle.

10.13 Setting Realistic Expectations

Unrealistic expectations often fuel stress and fear. If you set the bar too high—whether at work, school, or in personal goals—you may constantly feel inadequate. Instead:

1. **Know Your Limits**: Everyone has a different capacity for tasks. Plan around your energy levels and resources.
2. **Celebrate Small Wins**: Recognize steps you complete instead of only celebrating major successes.
3. **Adjust Goals When Needed**: Life changes. Adapt your plans if a new situation arises—like health challenges or family duties.
4. **Avoid Comparing**: Each person's journey is unique. Comparing your progress to others can create unnecessary stress.

Realistic expectations help you work steadily without overwhelming yourself with impossible standards.

10.14 Combining Problem-Solving with Stress Relief

Stress often comes from unsolved problems. A two-part approach can help:

1. **Problem-Solving Mode**:
    - **Identify the Issue**: Define the problem clearly (e.g., "I can't pay my bills this month").
    - **Brainstorm Solutions**: List any possible fixes without judgment—cut expenses, ask for a payment plan, find a side job, etc.
    - **Choose and Act**: Pick the most feasible solution and take immediate steps.
2. **Stress Relief Mode**:
    - **Relaxation Techniques**: After problem-solving, do something calming, like taking a walk or listening to soothing music.
    - **Healthy Distraction**: Watch a comedy, read a novel, or spend time on a favorite hobby to shift your mood.
    - **Positive Self-Talk**: Remind yourself you are doing the best you can.

Balancing these two modes ensures you are both addressing the root issues and managing your emotional response.

10.15 Embracing Imperfection to Combat Fear

Many fears stem from the desire to be perfect—perfect job performance, perfect parenting, perfect appearance. This perfectionism is stressful:

1. **Redefine Success**: Success can be learning something new or making a small improvement. It does not have to mean flawless results.
2. **Learn from Mistakes**: Mistakes are not failures; they are data points showing what does not work. Use them to refine your approach.
3. **Practice Self-Compassion**: Speak kindly to yourself if things go wrong. "I tried my best, and I can try again" is better than "I messed up and I'm worthless."
4. **Applaud Effort**: Celebrate effort as much as achievement. Consistent effort, even when results are slow, builds resilience.

Letting go of the idea of perfection frees you to take risks and reduces the fear of not being "enough."

10.16 When Professional Help Is Needed

Sometimes self-help methods are not sufficient. Certain signs indicate that it might be time to consult a professional:

- **Ongoing Symptoms**: If severe anxiety, panic, or depression persists for weeks or months despite your best efforts.
- **Daily Life Disruption**: When you cannot work, maintain relationships, or perform normal tasks because of fear or stress.
- **Physical Health Decline**: Constant stress leading to frequent illnesses, extreme fatigue, or chronic pain.
- **Thoughts of Harm**: If you ever feel hopeless or consider harming yourself or others, seek immediate help from a mental health crisis line or emergency services.

Therapists, psychologists, or psychiatrists are trained to provide specialized support. Treatment might include counseling, medication, or tailored strategies to help you regain control.

10.17 Building Emotional Resilience Alongside Stress Management

Earlier chapters discussed emotional resilience. Pairing resilience with stress management creates a robust approach:

1. **Flexible Mindset**: Stress is easier to handle when you adapt quickly to changes and setbacks.
2. **Healthy Outlets**: Have go-to hobbies or people you can turn to for release.
3. **Regular Reflection**: Periodically review your stress levels, what triggered them, and how you handled them. Learn and adjust.
4. **Gratitude**: Focusing on what you do have can temper feelings of scarcity or fear. Try a daily gratitude journal.
5. **Self-Efficacy**: Recognize that you have tackled problems before. This proof of past success can give you the strength to face new challenges.

A resilient mindset acknowledges difficulties but refuses to let them define your entire perspective.

10.18 Real-Life Example: Carmen's Story

Carmen was juggling two jobs and caring for her teenage daughter. She constantly worried she would fail at everything—paying the bills, being a good mom, keeping up with friends. Her stress was so intense that she hardly slept. Exhausted and on the edge of burnout, Carmen decided to make changes.

She started small: each morning, she spent five minutes practicing deep breathing and writing one thing she was grateful for (often her supportive sister or a good meal she had). She realized much of her fear was tied to an inability to manage her time. So she began using a monthly calendar, marking work shifts, her daughter's events, and her own downtime. Even a simple hour-long break on Sunday afternoon became a treasure for her mental well-being.

Additionally, Carmen talked to her daughter about sharing household chores. This eased her workload and gave her teenager more responsibility. She also joined a local parent support group, where she exchanged tips about budgeting and stress relief. Over a few months, Carmen felt lighter. Her problems did not vanish, but she learned coping strategies. Her sleepless nights decreased, she felt more organized, and the fear of "failing" lessened significantly. Carmen discovered that managing stress and fear is a process of steady, thoughtful steps.

10.19 Monitoring Your Progress and Adjusting

Managing fear and stress is not a one-time fix; it is an ongoing practice. Check in with yourself regularly:

- **Reduced Anxiety**: Are you feeling calmer overall? Do you recover from stressful events faster than before?
- **Improved Sleep**: Do you fall asleep more easily, or wake up feeling more rested?
- **Less Physical Tension**: Are aches, headaches, or stomach pains occurring less often?
- **Positive Outlook**: Have you noticed fewer catastrophic thoughts and more hopeful ones?
- **Better Time Management**: Are you meeting deadlines with less last-minute panic?

If you are not seeing improvements, tweak your techniques. Maybe you need more social support or a different relaxation method. Keep experimenting until you find a rhythm that works.

CHAPTER 11

Embracing Your Unique Qualities

11.1 Introduction: The Beauty of Individuality

Every person in this world has something that sets them apart—something unique that no one else can copy. It could be a special talent, a personal experience, or even a way of seeing the world. These unique qualities often shape how we interact with others, the goals we pursue, and the perspective we hold on life. Embracing what makes you different can feel both exciting and scary. Yet, when you accept and celebrate your individuality, you strengthen your sense of self and boost your confidence.

Some people spend years trying to blend in, believing it is safer or easier. While there is comfort in following the crowd, hiding your true self can lead to unhappiness or a sense of emptiness. True joy often comes from living authentically, which includes owning your quirks, talents, and personal style. This chapter will show you how to recognize and cherish your unique traits, break free from constant comparison, and let your individuality shine.

11.2 Why Your Unique Qualities Matter

When we talk about "unique qualities," we mean the traits, skills, experiences, or viewpoints that distinguish you from others. These qualities can come from your cultural background, personal struggles, passions, hobbies, or any number of factors. So why do they matter?

1. **They Shape Your Perspective**
   The way you see the world is different from anyone else. Your experiences combine in a special way to guide your thoughts and decisions. This unique perspective can help you solve problems creatively and approach situations with fresh ideas.
2. **They Contribute to Group Diversity**
   In teams—be it at work, in a community group, or even within a

family—diverse viewpoints often lead to better solutions. Embracing your individuality can spark valuable insights that others might never consider.
3. **They Foster Self-Discovery**
   Understanding your distinctive strengths and interests helps you grow. You learn what excites you, what troubles you, and where you can excel. This self-discovery paves the way for deeper confidence.
4. **They Make Life More Interesting**
   A world where everyone acts, thinks, and looks the same would be dull. Our differences add color and richness to life, leading to art, music, literature, and innovations we might not have otherwise.

By valuing your unique qualities, you not only honor yourself, but also enrich those around you.

11.3 Identifying Your Unique Qualities

For some people, it is immediately clear: maybe they have a rare artistic skill or a remarkable story of overcoming an obstacle. For others, their distinct traits can feel subtle or hidden. Here are practical ways to uncover what sets you apart:

1. **Reflect on Your Childhood**
   Think back to what you loved doing as a child. Did you enjoy building things with your hands? Were you a natural storyteller? Sometimes, childhood passions point to innate gifts or traits.
2. **Ask for Feedback**
   Friends, family members, or mentors might notice qualities in you that you take for granted. For instance, they may see you as unusually patient, or they might admire your sense of humor.
3. **Examine Your Challenges**
   Often, our struggles shape us in unique ways. Going through a health condition or dealing with a family crisis can give you empathy, strength, or insight that others might not have.
4. **Spot Your Sparks**
   Pay attention to moments when your eyes light up, your heart beats faster, or you lose track of time. These "sparks" might indicate a deep passion or talent.

5. **Journal Regularly**
   Writing down your daily thoughts can reveal patterns in your interests and values. Over time, you will see which topics you return to and why they fascinate you.

By consistently exploring these areas, you gradually form a clearer picture of the special qualities that define you.

11.4 Overcoming the Pressure to Conform

In many cultures, there is pressure to fit a certain mold—whether it is tied to appearance, career choices, or life milestones. This can cause us to hide our individuality. You might think, "If I do not follow the crowd, people will judge me," or "I have to look and act like everyone else to succeed." While it is true that society often has expectations, it is also true that some of the most successful and admired individuals stepped outside common norms.

- **Recognize Your Fears**: Make a list of what you are worried will happen if you show your real self. Are you afraid of rejection, criticism, or feeling awkward?
- **Question Those Fears**: Ask yourself, "Is this fear based on fact or assumption?" In many cases, we overestimate negative outcomes.
- **Look for Role Models**: Identify people you admire for their uniqueness. How did they handle societal pressure? Often, they stood firm in their identity, and it paved the way for their success.
- **Celebrate Small Acts of Individuality**: Start with small steps—wear a piece of clothing that represents your style or share an unusual hobby with a friend. These small acts build your comfort level over time.

Conforming can be useful in certain contexts, like following workplace rules or respecting cultural traditions. But completely hiding who you are can lead to ongoing tension. Learning to find a balance between respect for community and personal expression can help you thrive.

11.5 The Comparison Trap and How to Break Free

Comparing yourself to others is one of the quickest ways to undermine your unique qualities. With social media, it can feel like everyone else is more talented, successful, or attractive. However, these comparisons are often based on incomplete information. People usually share only their best moments online, not the behind-the-scenes struggles.

Steps to Avoid the Comparison Trap:

1. **Limit Social Media**: If scrolling through your feeds leaves you feeling inadequate, reduce your time online or unfollow accounts that trigger negative thoughts.
2. **Focus on Growth, Not Perfection**: Everyone has different starting points and personal journeys. Instead of "I am not as good as her," think, "I can improve by learning from her approach."
3. **Track Your Progress**: Keep a journal or list of your personal wins and lessons learned. Reviewing these entries can remind you how far you have come.
4. **Gratitude Practice**: Write down a few things you are grateful for each day, including aspects of yourself. This habit helps shift attention from what you lack to what you already have.

Remind yourself that your path is yours alone. The successes or struggles of others do not diminish your worth. Indeed, there is plenty of room for all of us to shine in different ways.

11.6 Nurturing Your Individual Style

Your unique qualities often show up in how you dress, the words you choose, the music you like, or the hobbies you pursue. Rather than fighting these instincts, nurture them. Below are a few ways:

1. **Experiment with Fashion**: Clothes can be a form of self-expression. Try new colors, patterns, or accessories that reflect your personality. You do not have to follow every trend—pick what resonates with you.
2. **Curate Your Space**: Whether it is your bedroom or a home office, decorate it with items that inspire you—a vision board, framed

artwork, or meaningful souvenirs. This personal environment can fuel creativity and remind you of who you are.
3. **Develop Unique Hobbies**: If you are curious about an activity—like pottery, salsa dancing, or coding—give it a try. Even if it is not a mainstream interest, exploring lesser-known hobbies can bring unexpected joy and new connections.
4. **Share Your Passions**: Do not hide what you love. Talk about your interests with friends or post updates about them online. You might find others who share your passion, leading to supportive friendships.
5. **Embrace Personal Rituals**: Maybe you love reading poetry every morning or walking in nature on weekends. These rituals can keep you connected to your authentic self amidst life's demands.

Letting your style and preferences evolve over time is natural. The key is to remain true to what genuinely excites and comforts you, rather than forcing a persona just to fit in.

11.7 Finding Confidence in Your Background and Culture

For many women, cultural or family background heavily shapes their identity. However, if you come from a minority culture or a family with certain expectations, you may feel torn between your heritage and the mainstream world. Instead of seeing your background as a barrier, try to view it as a treasure chest of traditions, languages, or experiences that enrich you.

1. **Learn Your Roots**: Educate yourself about your family history or cultural heritage. This knowledge can boost pride and connection.
2. **Fuse Old and New**: Look for ways to blend traditional elements with modern life. This might mean cooking dishes from your culture while also exploring global recipes.
3. **Share Stories**: Talk to family elders, gather stories or recipes, and pass them on. Each generation adds its own layer, making your identity richer.
4. **Use Your Bilingual Skills**: If you speak more than one language, celebrate this advantage. Being bilingual can open up career paths, enhance travel experiences, and help you connect with diverse communities.

By integrating your background into your daily life, you can stand tall knowing you are part of a larger story. This sense of belonging can enhance your self-esteem and remind you that your uniqueness is partly shaped by those who came before you.

11.8 Turning Past Pain into Strength

Life's challenges can leave emotional scars. Perhaps you have gone through a difficult breakup, lost a loved one, struggled with health issues, or faced discrimination. Though painful, these experiences can be part of what makes you uniquely strong or compassionate. The key is learning to process the pain and transform it into something positive.

- **Acknowledge Your Feelings**: Instead of ignoring or minimizing your hurt, allow yourself time to grieve or be angry. Journaling, therapy, or talking to a trusted friend can help.
- **Extract Lessons**: Ask yourself, "What did this teach me about my values, my limits, or my resilience?" Pain often pushes us to grow in ways we would not otherwise.
- **Find Purpose**: Some people turn their struggles into a mission—like volunteering, mentoring, or starting a community project. This focus can give new meaning to past hardships.
- **Celebrate Survivorship**: If you have overcome a serious obstacle, remember to acknowledge that victory. Whether it is sobriety, healing from trauma, or stepping away from toxic situations, these achievements are part of your unique identity.

Each time you conquer a challenge, you add a layer of depth to who you are. Embracing these layers makes you more compassionate toward yourself and others.

11.9 Learning to Accept Praise and Recognition

Many women feel uneasy when complimented. They may brush it off or downplay their accomplishments: "Oh, it was nothing." Over time, this can send a message to your own mind (and others) that you do not value your *unique abilities. Learning to accept praise is a key step in embracing who you are.*

1. **Say "Thank You"**: *A simple "thank you" acknowledges the compliment without argument or dismissal.*
2. **Avoid Self-Deprecating Remarks**: *Instead of answering a compliment with, "I messed up a lot, though," try, "I appreciate that. I worked hard on it."*
3. **Reflect on the Compliment**: *Later, think about what the praise might mean. Are you truly skilled at comforting friends? Did you really do an excellent job on a work project? Let yourself believe it.*
4. **Pay It Forward**: *Giving sincere compliments to others can help you feel more comfortable receiving them, too. Recognizing someone else's unique traits fosters a cycle of positive support.*

Allowing praise does not make you arrogant. It helps reinforce a healthy self-image and reminds you that your unique contributions matter.

11.10 Real-Life Example: Mira's Authentic Transformation

Mira grew up in a family that valued quiet obedience. She was shy and rarely voiced her opinions. During college, she discovered a love for spoken word poetry. At first, she was terrified to perform, but she felt a deep pull to share her words. She started attending small poetry nights. Her voice shook, and her palms were sweaty, but she poured her emotions into each piece.

Over time, Mira realized her poems connected with others. People praised her courage and unique style, describing her lines as raw and stirring. Despite her trembling voice, she learned to accept that these performances captured what she saw as flaws—her shy nature and her intense feelings—and turned them into art. She embraced her gentle voice and personal experiences. Soon, she led a campus group for aspiring poets, teaching them how to find their own voices.

Mira's life changed because she dared to celebrate her unique qualities. She no longer apologized for being sensitive or quiet. Instead, she channeled these traits into a creative strength. Her story reminds us that stepping into your authenticity can open doors you never even knew existed.

11.11 Practical Exercises to Embrace Your Uniqueness

1. **Create a "Brag Sheet"**
   List your positive traits, accomplishments, and things you love about yourself. Read it whenever you feel inadequate.
2. **Design a Personal Logo or Motto**
   If you had to represent yourself with a simple symbol or phrase, what would it be? Drawing or writing it out can help you clarify who you are at your core.
3. **Weekly Reflection**
   At the end of each week, write down one thing that felt authentically you—maybe wearing an outfit that showed your style, or speaking your mind in a meeting. Notice how it felt.
4. **Attempt Something Outside Your Comfort Zone**
   This should be something that aligns with your hidden interests or talents, like signing up for a comedy open mic or painting class. Document how you feel before and after.
5. **Self-Interview**
   Imagine you are a journalist asking yourself questions about your life story, struggles, and dreams. Answer honestly in writing or out loud. This creative approach can reveal surprising insights.

11.12 Building Supportive Connections

Part of embracing your uniqueness is finding people who appreciate you for who you are. While not everyone will celebrate your individuality, nurturing relationships that do can boost your confidence.

- **Seek Like-Minded Communities**: Join clubs, online forums, or local groups that share your interests or values.
- **Avoid Toxic Relationships**: If people constantly belittle or ignore your unique traits, consider whether you need to limit your time with them.
- **Be Open About Your Passions**: When you share your excitement with others, you might attract those who resonate with it.

- **Offer Encouragement**: Show genuine interest in what makes others unique, too. This reciprocity strengthens bonds and fosters mutual support.

Surrounding yourself with positive influences can reinforce that it is safe and rewarding to be exactly who you are.

11.13 Balancing Individuality with Teamwork

Sometimes people worry that emphasizing their unique qualities might isolate them from group activities. But in truth, being authentic can strengthen teams. When each member embraces their distinct strengths, a group can tackle challenges more effectively. Still, collaboration requires respect for others' viewpoints.

- **Clearly Define Roles**: If you have a special skill—like organizing events—take the lead in that area. Allow teammates to shine in their fields as well.
- **Communicate**: Explain why you hold certain opinions or approaches. This transparency makes it easier for others to see the value of your perspective.
- **Stay Flexible**: Embracing your uniqueness should not mean dismissing others. Listen to diverse inputs and adapt when it benefits the group goal.
- **Celebrate Team Achievements**: Applaud collective efforts while acknowledging individual contributions. Everyone feels valued, including you.

When you show up as yourself and respect the uniqueness of others, you create a richer, more functional environment for all.

11.14 Dealing with Criticism or Mockery

Not everyone will applaud your individuality. Some people might tease or criticize you for being different. This can sting, but it does not have to derail your self-confidence.

1. **Separate Constructive Feedback from Teasing**: If someone offers a thoughtful critique—like suggesting ways to improve your skill—listen. But if they simply mock you, recognize that it reflects more on them than on you.
2. **Respond Calmly**: Getting defensive or angry might escalate things. A simple statement like, "I understand you see it differently, but I'm comfortable with who I am," can end the conversation gracefully.
3. **Find Allies**: If you frequently face negativity, confide in supportive friends or mentors. They can remind you why your uniqueness matters.
4. **Stand Firm**: If a situation becomes hostile or abusive, consider removing yourself from it. Your well-being is worth more than any attempt to please unkind people.

Criticism can be an opportunity to reaffirm your sense of self. You are not defined by others' narrow views.

11.15 Embracing Growth and Change

Your unique qualities do not have to remain static. As you explore life, you might discover new passions or realize old patterns no longer serve you. Embracing change is also part of authenticity.

- **Regular Self-Check-Ins**: Periodically ask, "Have my interests or values shifted? Am I clinging to a past identity out of habit?"
- **Stay Curious**: Try new experiences without worrying if they match your previous preferences. Growth often comes from exploring unfamiliar paths.
- **Allow Yourself to Evolve**: You might go through a season of life where you focus on a certain skill, only to shift gears later. That is okay; evolution is natural.
- **Communicate Changes**: If you have friends or family who knew "old you," share why you have changed. Explain your new interests or viewpoints so they understand and can support you.

Authenticity does not mean staying the same forever. It means being honest about who you are in each phase of your journey.

11.16 How Embracing Uniqueness Builds Confidence

When you celebrate your distinct qualities, you become more comfortable in your own skin. This comfort fuels self-assurance. You no longer feel as compelled to hide or apologize for what sets you apart. Instead, you might even showcase it, whether at work, in social settings, or online. Over time, this sense of ownership and pride in who you are seeps into everything you do, from how you speak to the risks you are willing to take. Confidence grows naturally from living in alignment with your true self.

Additionally, embracing your individuality can help you cope better with rejection or failure. When you stand firm in your own identity, you understand that a setback in one area does not define your entire worth. You can move forward, learning from the experience while keeping your self-esteem intact.

11.17 Realigning After Self-Doubt

Even the most self-assured people have moments of doubt. You might catch yourself comparing again or feel uncertain about your choices. When that happens:

1. **Pause**: *Recognize the self-doubt and label it as a temporary feeling.*
2. **Review Past Successes**: *Remind yourself of times you stood out in a good way or overcame fears by being yourself.*
3. **Seek Encouragement**: *Talk to a trusted friend, mentor, or therapist who supports your personal growth.*
4. **Take a Break**: *Sometimes, simply stepping away from the stressful environment—like social media or certain peer groups—can help you regain perspective.*
5. **Practice a Grounding Ritual**: *Perform a short relaxation or breathing exercise to center yourself. Then ask, "What do I truly want?" This question can refocus you on your authentic desires.*

Self-doubt may never vanish completely, but learning to address it quickly stops it from overshadowing your unique qualities.

11.18 Benefits of a Strong Sense of Individuality

By fully embracing your uniqueness, you can experience several long-term benefits:

- **Personal Fulfillment**: You live a life that aligns with your true nature, reducing the stress of pretending to be someone else.
- **Better Decision-Making**: Knowing who you are clarifies your values, making it easier to choose paths that fit your goals.
- **Positive Influence**: When others see you being comfortable in your own skin, they might feel inspired to do the same.
- **Creative Expression**: Authentic living often fuels creativity. You may find fresh ideas for projects, art, or solutions to everyday problems.
- **Resilience**: Holding onto your individuality can help you bounce back when facing challenges, because you trust your inner compass.

These outcomes not only benefit you but also resonate with friends, family, and the wider community who appreciate genuine connections.

11.19 Supporting Others in Their Uniqueness

A key part of embracing your individuality is respecting others' uniqueness too. You can foster a supportive environment by:

- **Practicing Non-Judgment**: Accept that people have different backgrounds, styles, and choices. That is part of what makes the world interesting.
- **Offering Encouragement**: If you see someone trying something new or standing out from the crowd, let them know you admire their courage.
- **Sharing Resources**: Recommend books, videos, or events that can help someone explore their interests.
- **Collaborating**: Find ways to combine your unique skills with theirs, creating something meaningful together.
- **Staying Open to Learning**: The more you engage with different perspectives, the more you grow and expand your own understanding.

When you uplift others in being themselves, you further affirm your own journey toward self-acceptance. It becomes a positive, reciprocal cycle.

CHAPTER 12

Building Positive Habits

12.1 Introduction: The Power of Habits

Habits are the small, repeated actions that shape much of our daily life. They can be as simple as the way you brush your teeth each morning or as big as how you approach your work tasks. Because habits are done automatically, they have the power to either propel us toward our goals or hold us back. Building positive habits—such as regular exercise, kind communication, or consistent self-care—can create a strong foundation for overall well-being and success.

Yet, forming new habits or breaking old ones is not always easy. You might start with enthusiasm but lose interest after a few days. Or you could feel overwhelmed by how many changes you want to make all at once. This chapter explores practical strategies for creating habits that stick. You will learn how to set realistic goals, overcome obstacles, and celebrate small wins so you can maintain momentum over the long haul.

12.2 Why Habits Are Crucial for Women's Confidence

Women often juggle multiple responsibilities—jobs, family, relationships, community duties, and personal aspirations. Good habits can reduce the stress of this balancing act. For example, if you develop a habit of setting aside 30 minutes each day for a specific task (like journaling or planning meals), you free up mental energy for other matters. You do not have to constantly decide if or when you will do it—your habit leads the way.

Positive habits also boost self-esteem. Each time you follow through on a commitment to yourself, you reinforce the belief that you are capable of reaching your goals. Over time, these small, repetitive successes add up, building a core sense of self-trust and accomplishment.

12.3 Understanding How Habits Form

Psychologists and behavioral experts often describe habit formation as a loop:

1. **Cue**: This is the trigger that signals your brain to start the habit. It could be a time of day, a location, a feeling, or an event.
2. **Routine**: The action you take automatically, such as brewing coffee first thing in the morning or checking your phone when you hear a notification.
3. **Reward**: The benefit or satisfaction you get from the habit. It might be the taste of coffee, the relief of stress, or the pleasure of connecting with friends on social media.

Over time, your brain starts to associate the cue with the routine and the reward. If the reward is positive, you are more likely to repeat the behavior. To build a new habit, you can consciously design or reshape these three components to work in your favor.

12.4 Identifying Which Habits to Build

You might have a long list of changes you want to make—waking up earlier, drinking more water, meditating, exercising, reading, learning a new language, and so on. While enthusiasm is great, trying to tackle too many habits at once can be overwhelming. Instead, prioritize:

1. **Pick One or Two**: Start with the habits that will have the biggest positive effect on your life. Maybe you want to improve your health first by walking daily and drinking enough water.
2. **Be Specific**: Rather than saying, "I want to be healthier," define a clear action: "I will walk for 20 minutes every weekday at 7:00 a.m."
3. **Consider Your Values**: Align your habit goals with what truly matters to you. If you value creativity, a daily habit of writing or painting might be more motivating than forcing yourself to read about financial markets (unless finance is also a genuine interest).
4. **Think Long-Term**: Choose habits you can see yourself maintaining beyond a short burst. A slow, steady approach often leads to lasting success.

Focusing on a few well-chosen habits builds a strong foundation, making it easier to add more positive changes later.

12.5 Setting Realistic and Measurable Goals

To turn a habit into a lasting part of your routine, you need clear, achievable targets. The well-known "SMART" framework can help:

- **Specific**: Define the action plainly: "Drink 8 cups of water daily," not just "Stay hydrated."
- **Measurable**: Track your progress. You could mark each glass of water on a sticky note or use a mobile app.
- **Achievable**: Start with a goal that fits your current lifestyle. If you are new to working out, 20 minutes of gentle exercise may be more realistic than running 5 miles every morning.
- **Relevant**: Pick habits that matter to you personally. A habit is harder to maintain if it is only based on external pressure from friends or media.
- **Time-Bound**: Decide on a timeframe. For instance, "I will follow this plan for the next 4 weeks," so you have a clear period to measure and evaluate success.

When you meet these criteria, your goals become easier to stick to because you know exactly what you are aiming for.

12.6 Overcoming Common Obstacles

Several barriers can disrupt your new habit-forming efforts:

1. **Lack of Motivation**
   - **Solution**: Remind yourself why this habit is important. Pair it with a short-term reward (like a favorite healthy snack after exercising) or a larger vision (like having more energy for your kids).
2. **Time Constraints**
   - **Solution**: Fit the habit into an existing routine. For example, do a short meditation right after brushing your teeth. Also

consider if you can delegate tasks or reorganize your schedule to carve out time.
3. **Stress and Fatigue**
    - **Solution**: Start small so the habit does not feel like a burden. Doing a 5-minute activity is better than skipping it entirely because you are tired.
4. **Negative Self-Talk**
    - **Solution**: Replace thoughts like "I will never stick to this" with "I am learning something new, and each attempt helps me grow." Seek encouragement from friends or mentors when self-doubt arises.
5. **Lack of Immediate Results**
    - **Solution**: Understand that habits often show cumulative benefits. Try to enjoy the process rather than expecting an overnight transformation.

By anticipating these challenges, you can create strategies to handle them before they derail your progress.

12.7 Linking Habits for Greater Success

A technique called "habit stacking" involves adding a new habit to something you already do consistently. For example:

- **After I brew my morning coffee (existing habit), I will write in my journal for 5 minutes (new habit).**
- **When I start my lunch break (existing habit), I will take a quick walk outside (new habit).**

By pairing your new habit with an established one, you create a natural cue that reminds you to perform the action. This approach makes it easier to remember and stick to the routine over time.

12.8 Using Accountability for Habit Formation

Accountability means being answerable to someone or something beyond yourself. It is a powerful motivator for maintaining new habits. Here are ways to set up accountability:

1. **Find a Partner**: Team up with a friend who has similar goals. If you both want to read more, agree to send each other quick updates or discuss a chapter weekly.
2. **Join a Group**: Many online forums or local clubs exist for fitness, writing, coding, and more. Sharing your progress with others can keep you on track.
3. **Hire a Coach**: A personal trainer, life coach, or mentor can provide expert guidance and expect regular check-ins.
4. **Public Commitments**: Declare your goal publicly, perhaps on social media or within a supportive community. Knowing others are watching can boost your discipline.
5. **Apps and Tools**: Some mobile apps gamify the habit-building process. They might reward you with badges for each day you complete a task, or send reminders when you skip it.

Accountability does not have to be stressful or rigid. It is simply an extra layer of support that helps you follow through on your intentions.

12.9 Celebrating Small Wins

One reason many people drop new habits is that they do not see immediate huge results. However, each small step is an accomplishment. Recognizing these micro-successes can keep you excited about the journey:

- **Track Your Streak**: Mark every day you follow your habit on a calendar or app. Seeing a chain of checked-off days motivates you to keep it unbroken.
- **Give Yourself Mini-Rewards**: After a week of consistent practice, treat yourself to something you enjoy—like a special coffee drink or a relaxing bath.

- **Acknowledge Growth**: Notice improvements, no matter how small. Maybe you feel a bit more flexible after daily stretches or slightly less stressed after a week of journaling.
- **Share Achievements**: If it is comfortable, tell a supportive friend or group. Hearing "well done" from others can reinforce your pride in progress.

By celebrating small wins, you nurture a positive mindset, which is essential for long-term habit success.

12.10 Tracking Progress and Adjusting Goals

Monitoring your habit-building journey helps you notice patterns and identify when you might need to tweak your plan. Some methods include:

1. **Daily or Weekly Log**
    - **What to Record**: Whether you completed the habit, how you felt, any problems you encountered.
    - **Benefit**: This fosters awareness and accountability.
2. **Visual Charts**
    - **What to Use**: Graphs, habit-tracking apps, or even a simple sticker chart on your fridge.
    - **Benefit**: Seeing a visual representation of your success can be highly motivating.
3. **Periodic Reviews**
    - **What to Ask**: "Is this habit still meaningful?" "Is the frequency right, or do I need to change it?" "Am I bored, or do I need a new challenge?"
    - **Benefit**: Keeps your habits fresh and aligned with your evolving life circumstances.

If you find your original goal is too easy, scale it up a bit. If it is too hard, simplify it. The ability to adapt ensures that your habit remains achievable and relevant.

12.11 Balancing Multiple Habits

Eventually, you may want to maintain several positive habits—like healthy eating, daily journaling, and regular exercise. Balancing them is possible if you:

1. **Introduce Them One by One**
   Start with a single habit. After it becomes comfortable, add a second habit, and so on. Avoid making huge lifestyle changes all at once, which can lead to burnout.
2. **Schedule Strategically**
   Plan specific times for each habit. For example, do a morning jog, an afternoon gratitude list, and an evening reading session.
3. **Keep Some Habits Very Small**
   Not every habit needs to be a major time commitment. Some can be micro-habits, like doing one yoga pose when you wake up or writing three bullet points in a journal.
4. **Check for Conflicts**
   Ensure your habits do not clash. If you plan to exercise at 7:00 p.m. but also want to have dinner with your family at that time, you will need to adjust.

Balancing habits is like spinning plates: it requires practice to keep them all in motion without dropping one.

12.12 The Role of Environment in Habit Building

Your surroundings heavily influence your actions, often in subtle ways. If you want to watch less TV but place your couch directly in front of a big screen, that environment cues you to watch. On the other hand, if you want to practice guitar, keeping it on a stand in plain sight can remind you to play.

- **Design Your Space**: Make healthy choices easy. Store fruits and vegetables at eye level. Put workout clothes where you will see them first thing in the morning.
- **Remove Temptations**: If you aim to reduce sugar, keep fewer sweets at home. If you want to read more, place your favorite book near your bed instead of your smartphone.

- **Use Positive Triggers**: Surround your desk with motivational quotes or place a sticky note with your habit goal on the bathroom mirror.
- **Align with Supportive People**: Spend time with individuals who share similar positive habits. Their environment becomes a strong influence, too.

When your space and social circle support your habits, the path to consistency becomes smoother.

12.13 Mindset Shifts for Lasting Habits

Sometimes, habits fail because we see them as temporary chores. Transforming them into part of your identity creates a stronger bond with the action:

1. **Identify as the Type of Person**: Instead of saying, "I want to run daily," say, "I am a runner." This subtle change influences choices—runners plan routes or invest in good shoes because that is what they do.
2. **Embrace Long-Term Thinking**: Picture yourself 1, 5, or 10 years from now, continuously practicing this habit. This visualization can motivate you to push past short-term inconveniences.
3. **Practice Self-Compassion**: Slip-ups happen. Missing a day or two does not mean you have failed. Accept the mistake, learn from it, and keep going without harsh self-blame.
4. **Stay Curious**: When challenges arise, ask, "Why did this happen, and how can I prevent it next time?" This approach turns obstacles into learning experiences rather than sources of frustration.

When you see your habits as part of who you are, maintaining them feels less forced and more natural.

12.14 Habit-Building and Stress Management

Building habits when life is calm is one thing; doing so under stress is another. However, consistent routines can actually help reduce stress because they bring structure and predictability to chaotic times.

- **Keep It Simple**: During stressful periods, do not overhaul every aspect of your life. Maintain just a few key habits (like a 5-minute daily stretch).
- **Use Habits as Anchors**: When everything else seems uncertain, turning to a familiar, positive routine can ground you emotionally.
- **Be Flexible**: If you cannot complete a 30-minute workout, do 10 minutes. Adapting your habit in tough times is better than abandoning it entirely.
- **Seek Support**: Let friends or family know you are trying to maintain habits under pressure. They may offer help or at least encouragement.

Habits can act as a supportive backbone, helping you navigate the storms of life without losing your sense of stability.

12.15 Real-Life Example: Tina's Habit Evolution

Tina wanted to improve her health but found it difficult to exercise regularly. She tried forcing herself to run 5 kilometers every morning, but after a week, she was exhausted and sore. She gave up, believing she "just wasn't disciplined." Then she decided to start smaller.

She set a goal: **walk for 10 minutes each day at 6:00 p.m.** She placed her walking shoes by the front door as a cue. After each walk, she allowed herself a few minutes of sitting on her porch, enjoying the view, as a reward. Within a month, walking for 10 minutes became a normal part of her day. Encouraged, she increased it to 20 minutes. She also discovered she felt more relaxed after walking, which motivated her further.

After six months, Tina was walking 30 minutes most evenings, had more energy, and even lost some weight. Inspired by her success, she began another habit—drinking more water. She used the same approach: a clear goal, a visual cue (a water bottle on her desk), and a simple reward (a sticker on her calendar each day she hit 8 cups). Tina's story shows how starting small and staying consistent can transform your lifestyle, one habit at a time.

12.16 Breaking Unhelpful Habits

Not all habits are positive. Some, like snacking too much on junk food, constantly checking your phone, or staying up too late, can undermine your well-being. Breaking these habits requires a reverse approach:

1. **Identify the Cue**: Notice what triggers the unwanted habit. Is it stress, boredom, or a certain time of day?
2. **Interrupt the Routine**: When you feel the urge, pause. Can you replace the action with a healthier alternative? For instance, if you snack when bored, do a quick puzzle or stretch instead.
3. **Change the Environment**: Make the unhealthy habit less convenient. Hide snacks in a hard-to-reach place, or turn off app notifications to reduce mindless phone use.
4. **Reward Positive Change**: Celebrate each time you resist the old habit. Over time, your brain will stop craving it as strongly if you consistently block its routine.
5. **Track Setbacks**: If you slip, note why it happened. Adjust your plan to avoid similar triggers in the future.

Breaking a habit can be challenging, but applying these steps gradually weakens its hold.

12.17 The Impact of Positive Habits on Self-Worth

When you keep promises to yourself, you affirm your own reliability and capacity to grow. Every time you say "I will do X" and then actually do it, you reinforce your self-trust. This shift in self-perception is powerful:

- **Greater Self-Confidence**: Knowing you can stick to your intentions shows you are capable of self-discipline and self-care.
- **Improved Mood**: Positive habits that involve health or creativity often have an uplifting effect, reducing anxiety or depressive feelings.
- **Better Boundaries**: As you spend time on beneficial routines, you learn to say no to distractions or obligations that do not align with your priorities.
- **Long-Term Success**: Habit mastery can spill over into professional achievements, healthier relationships, and a balanced lifestyle.

Over time, the effect multiplies. One positive habit can spark a chain reaction, leading you to tackle bigger challenges with confidence.

12.18 Reevaluating and Renewing Habits Over Time

Life is not static. As your schedule, interests, or health change, certain habits may need to be retired or modified:

- **Regular Check-Ins**: Every few months, review your routines. Do they still serve your current goals or circumstances?
- **Adapt Gradually**: If you used to do a 60-minute workout but now have a busier schedule, a 20-minute workout might be more realistic.
- **Stay Open**: Be willing to explore new habits if your passions shift. Maybe you become interested in gardening or cooking. Embrace fresh routines as you grow.

By updating your habits to match the flow of your life, you prevent boredom and keep your routines aligned with what truly matters.

12.19 Supporting Others in Building Habits

Helping friends or family form positive habits can also strengthen your own commitment. Here's how:

- **Offer Encouragement**: Send quick messages of support when they meet their daily goal.
- **Be a Role Model**: Let them see you maintaining your habits. This can inspire them to stay consistent, too.
- **Share Resources**: Recommend apps, books, or articles about habit-building.
- **Avoid Nagging**: Gentle reminders can be helpful, but constant pushing can backfire. Let them set their own pace.

When you foster a community of mutual support, everyone benefits from shared motivation and accountability.

CHAPTER 13

Relationships and Social Support

13.1 Introduction: Humans Are Social Beings

No matter how independent we try to be, we all rely on social connections in one way or another. Whether it is leaning on a friend for advice, sharing laughter with family, or collaborating with coworkers, healthy relationships can add richness and balance to our lives. For women, in particular, social bonds often play a big role in building emotional well-being and resilience.

This chapter explores the importance of strong relationships and social support in everyday life. We will look at how to create new friendships, nurture existing bonds, and cope with conflict in a constructive manner. By understanding what makes a supportive connection, you can become more intentional about forming and maintaining healthy relationships. Strong social support not only helps you navigate challenges, it also inspires confidence, enhances happiness, and opens you up to new possibilities.

13.2 Why Relationships Matter for Women's Confidence

It is easier to feel confident when you know that someone has your back. Whether it is a best friend, a mentor, or a loving partner, a caring support system can provide encouragement, guidance, and reassurance. Feeling understood and accepted can counteract self-doubt and the fear of judgment. When you achieve a goal or face a setback, having people to celebrate or commiserate with can keep you motivated.

Conversely, loneliness or isolation can amplify insecurities. Without a support network, everyday stressors might appear overwhelming, making it harder to maintain self-belief. Feeling alone in your struggles might lead you to question your ability to handle life's ups and downs. By investing in relationships, you create a cushion that softens life's inevitable blows, allowing your confidence to remain intact even under pressure.

13.3 Recognizing Supportive Versus Toxic Connections

All relationships are not created equal. Some people genuinely uplift you, while others undermine you—intentionally or unintentionally. Identifying the difference between a supportive connection and a toxic one is crucial. Here are some signs to watch for:

Supportive Connections

- **Active Listening**: They pay attention when you speak, showing genuine interest.
- **Respect for Boundaries**: They honor your personal limits without pushing or manipulating you.
- **Encouragement**: They celebrate your wins and cheer you on, rather than feeling threatened by your success.
- **Constructive Feedback**: They offer insights or critiques that help you grow, rather than tearing you down.
- **Balance**: Both of you give and receive in the relationship, ensuring neither party feels used.

Toxic Connections

- **Constant Criticism**: They judge your choices harshly or belittle your achievements.
- **Manipulation**: They guilt-trip you into doing things or ignore your boundaries.
- **Jealousy or Envy**: They show little happiness for your successes, sometimes making snide remarks.
- **Emotional Drain**: You often leave interactions feeling stressed, anxious, or unhappy.
- **One-Sided Support**: They expect you to be there for them but offer little in return.

Sometimes a relationship is not entirely toxic but has unhealthy patterns that need addressing. It can help to talk openly and work together on changes. However, if someone repeatedly disrespects you, it might be time to limit or even end contact for the sake of your well-being.

13.4 Building and Expanding Your Social Circle

For many adults—especially women juggling jobs, family, or other obligations—finding new friends can seem daunting. Yet, social circles can shift over time, and making new connections can be both refreshing and empowering. Here are ways to build supportive relationships:

1. **Follow Your Interests**
    - **Why It Works**: When you join groups or events that match your passions—like a book club, cooking class, or hiking group—you meet people with similar hobbies. This shared interest can spark quick conversations and potential friendships.
    - **How to Start**: Look for local meetups, community classes, or online forums where you can connect over topics you genuinely enjoy.
2. **Volunteer or Get Involved in the Community**
    - **Why It Works**: Volunteering for a cause you believe in, such as a food bank, animal shelter, or community center, lets you meet like-minded individuals who care about similar issues.
    - **How to Start**: Check local community websites or social media groups for volunteer listings. Commit to a regular schedule if possible so you can build ongoing connections.
3. **Leverage Social Media Wisely**
    - **Why It Works**: While social media can be superficial if used aimlessly, it can also help you discover local events and groups that match your interests.
    - **How to Start**: Join relevant Facebook groups, follow local event pages, or consider apps designed for making new friends in your area.
4. **Reconnect with Old Acquaintances**
    - **Why It Works**: Sometimes past classmates or coworkers share similar life experiences. Reconnecting can rekindle a bond you once found meaningful.
    - **How to Start**: A simple message or phone call saying "I was thinking about you—how have you been?" can open the door to renewed friendship.

Remember, real friendship takes time to grow. Be patient, keep showing genuine interest in others, and do not be afraid to ask someone to grab coffee if you feel a spark of connection.

13.5 Maintaining Healthy Friendships and Family Ties

Once you have a circle of friends or close family members, the next step is to sustain those bonds in a healthy manner. That often requires consistent effort, patience, and understanding:

1. **Regular Communication**
     - **Phone or Video Calls**: Hearing a loved one's voice can create a stronger sense of closeness than text messages alone.
     - **Small Gestures**: Send a card or note on birthdays or significant anniversaries. Little moments of recognition show that you care.
2. **Setting Boundaries**
     - **Time and Emotional Limits**: Even close friends need some personal space. Communicate if you are unable to meet or need some quiet time.
     - **Respect Differences**: Friends or family may have values that differ from yours. Aim to accept those differences, as long as they do not conflict with your well-being.
3. **Quality Over Quantity**
     - **Deep Conversations**: Instead of daily small talk, occasional heart-to-heart chats can foster stronger connections.
     - **Shared Activities**: Doing things together—like cooking a meal or going on a nature walk—can refresh the bond and create new memories.
4. **Forgiveness and Understanding**
     - **Conflict Resolution**: When disagreements happen, approach them calmly. Use statements that start with "I feel..." rather than "You always..." to avoid blame.
     - **Repairing Damage**: If a misunderstanding arises, be willing to apologize or accept an apology. Holding grudges can strain relationships that are otherwise beneficial.

These practices ensure that your relationships remain sources of comfort and mutual growth rather than stress or confusion.

13.6 Finding Mentors and Role Models

Beyond friendships, having a mentor or a role model can significantly enrich your life. A mentor is someone experienced who offers guidance, while a role model is someone you look up to for inspiration—though you might not know them personally. Here is how they can help:

- **Career Advancement**: A professional mentor can offer insights into your field, helping you navigate challenges and set realistic goals.
- **Personal Growth**: Mentors or role models can demonstrate how they overcame obstacles, providing hope and strategies for your own path.
- **Confidence Boost**: Seeing someone you admire succeed can remind you that your dreams are achievable. Hearing their challenges can also humanize the journey, making it feel less intimidating.

To find a mentor, you might consider professional networks, alumni groups, or simply reaching out to someone you respect via a polite email. Role models can be found by reading biographies, following thought leaders online, or listening to interviews. Even if you do not communicate directly with them, observing their work and mindset can give you direction and inspiration.

13.7 Romantic Relationships and Emotional Support

Romantic partnerships can be a powerful form of social support when nurtured with respect, trust, and open communication. However, reliance on one romantic partner for all emotional needs can be overwhelming for both partners. It is healthy to balance a romantic relationship with friendships, family, and personal interests.

1. **Open Dialogue**
    - **Sharing Feelings**: Regularly talk about what is on your mind—your worries, hopes, and daily events. Listening and validating each other's experiences fosters closeness.

- **Conflict Management**: Use constructive language during disagreements. Instead of "You never understand me," say, "I feel hurt when we do not talk through our problems."
2. **Mutual Respect**
    - **Personal Boundaries**: Even in a close relationship, each person needs some alone time or privacy. Respect each other's personal space.
    - **Shared Decision-Making**: Consider both perspectives when making big life choices, whether it is finances, moving to a new place, or planning for the future.
3. **Encouragement**
    - **Career and Life Goals**: Support each other's ambitions, celebrating milestones and offering a shoulder during setbacks.
    - **Emotional Safety**: Aim to be each other's safe haven, where you can express worries without fear of judgment.

A healthy romantic relationship can significantly boost confidence and well-being, but it flourishes best within a wider support network that includes friends, family, and colleagues.

13.8 Navigating Workplace Relationships

Many of us spend a large portion of our time at work, so it makes sense that workplace relationships matter. Constructive relationships with colleagues can make your job more enjoyable, reduce stress, and even open doors for career advancement. To build productive professional connections:

1. **Be Friendly but Professional**
    - **Greeting and Courtesy**: A simple "good morning" or "hello" can set a positive tone. Listening attentively when colleagues speak indicates respect.
    - **Team Player**: Offer help when someone is overwhelmed, but be careful not to overpromise if your own workload is high.
2. **Communication**
    - **Clarity**: Whether through emails or face-to-face discussions, be clear about your ideas, deadlines, and expectations. Miscommunications can strain relationships.

- **Feedback Style**: When you need to give or receive feedback, approach it with a solution-focused attitude rather than mere criticism.

3. **Respect Differences**
     - **Diverse Work Styles**: Some people prefer brainstorming sessions, others like structured plans. Adapting and finding middle ground can increase team harmony.
     - **Cultural and Personal Backgrounds**: In a globalized environment, coworkers might have varied traditions or communication norms. Patience and open-mindedness go a long way.
4. **Handle Conflict Calmly**
     - **Avoid Gossip**: Talking behind someone's back rarely solves the issue and can create a toxic environment.
     - **Direct Conversation**: If tension arises, suggest a private talk to understand each other's viewpoints. Aim for a "win-win" outcome if possible.

Good workplace relationships can provide a sense of belonging and stability in a significant area of your life. They also foster a support network that may help you navigate career decisions or challenges.

13.9 Dealing with Social Anxiety

Not everyone feels confident in social situations. If you experience social anxiety or extreme shyness, forming relationships might be challenging. Yet, social support is still critical, and there are ways to overcome nervousness in group settings:

1. **Start Small**
     - **One-on-One**: It might feel less intimidating to meet people individually rather than in large gatherings.
     - **Familiar Settings**: Choose places you feel comfortable—like a quiet café or a park bench—so you are not overwhelmed by noise or crowds.
2. **Practice Gradually**
     - **Role-Play**: Rehearse conversations or greetings with a friend or family member. Simple practice can ease your anxiety.

- **Short Engagements**: Limit the time you spend at events. Plan to stay for half an hour and see how you feel, extending your stay if you become more relaxed.
3. **Therapy or Counseling**
   - **Professional Help**: Cognitive-behavioral therapy (CBT) or other forms of counseling can equip you with strategies to manage anxious thoughts.
   - **Support Groups**: Joining a group of people facing similar challenges can help you realize you are not alone.
4. **Mindset Shift**
   - **Focus on Learning**: Instead of judging each interaction as "good" or "bad," view social events as practice sessions.
   - **Celebrate Small Wins**: If you managed to talk to one new person or stayed longer than you usually would, that is progress.

Social anxiety can improve over time with consistent effort. You do not have to become an extrovert; you simply need to find comfort in connecting at your own pace.

13.10 Supporting Others While Maintaining Self-Care

Relationships are two-way streets. While you hope for support, you also want to offer kindness and empathy. However, there is a delicate balance. If you give too much—emotionally, physically, or financially—you risk burnout. Here's how to provide help while caring for yourself:

1. **Identify Your Limits**
   - **Emotional Boundaries**: Notice if you feel drained or resentful after constantly listening to a friend's problems. Politely suggest alternative resources or set time limits for venting sessions.
   - **Practical Boundaries**: If someone repeatedly asks for favors, decide what you can feasibly offer without neglecting your own responsibilities.
2. **Encourage Independence**

- **Empower Them**: Rather than solving every problem for someone, nudge them to explore their own solutions. This not only preserves your energy but also aids their personal growth.
- **Point to Resources**: If you are not qualified to handle a situation—like serious mental health concerns—help them find professional support.
3. **Check Your Motivations**
    - **Avoid "Fixing" Mode**: Sometimes, women feel compelled to rescue others. Ask yourself if you are stepping in because they truly cannot cope or because you feel obligated.
    - **Offer Genuine Care**: When you help from a place of compassion rather than guilt, it is more sustainable and healthy.

Balanced giving can strengthen your relationships without sacrificing your well-being or sense of self.

13.11 Creating Support Networks in Different Life Stages

Women often go through various life phases—school, career changes, marriage, motherhood, or caring for aging parents. Each stage can shift your social needs. Adapting your support network to fit your current reality is crucial:

1. **College or Early Career**
    - **Networking Events**: Attending career fairs or alumni gatherings can help you meet mentors and peers in your field.
    - **Campus Clubs**: Joining clubs or study groups can spark friendships that extend beyond graduation.
2. **Marriage or Long-Term Relationships**
    - **Couples' Communities**: Some areas have clubs or groups for couples, offering a chance to socialize and learn from others in similar relationship stages.
    - **Personal Hobbies**: Maintain your individual pursuits so you have a social circle outside the relationship as well.
3. **Parenthood**
    - **Parenting Groups**: Local community centers or online forums can connect you with other mothers facing similar challenges.

- **Family-Friendly Events**: Participate in playdates or family outings, where you can chat with other parents while the kids interact.
4. **Midlife and Beyond**
    - **Community Classes**: Art, fitness, or language classes can bring fresh social connections if your older friendships have drifted.
    - **Volunteer Work**: Contributing your time to meaningful causes often leads to friendships based on shared values.

Staying flexible and proactive in seeking out new groups ensures you remain socially fulfilled throughout changing life circumstances.

13.12 Overcoming Betrayal or Loss in Relationships

Unfortunately, not all relationships last. Some end through betrayal, and others fade due to changing paths. Dealing with this pain can be tough, but there are steps to help you move forward:

1. **Acknowledge the Hurt**
    - **Allow Emotions**: Give yourself permission to grieve, cry, or vent in a safe environment.
    - **Seek Support**: Talk to someone you trust—a friend, therapist, or support group.
2. **Reflect on the Lesson**
    - **Self-Inquiry**: Ask, "What can this teach me about my own boundaries or needs?"
    - **Avoid Self-Blame**: A failed relationship often involves multiple factors. Do not shoulder all responsibility if the other person acted dishonestly or aggressively.
3. **Focus on Healing**
    - **Self-Care**: Engage in activities that nurture your spirit, like nature walks, creative pursuits, or relaxation techniques.
    - **Gradual Rebuilding**: Over time, you may open yourself up to new friendships or partnerships. Proceed at a pace that feels right for you.
4. **Consider Professional Help**
    - **Counseling**: If you feel stuck or unable to move past the loss, therapy can provide tools for processing pain.

- **Support Groups**: Others who have gone through similar experiences may offer empathy and validation.

From heartbreak can come new understanding and stronger resilience. Allow yourself the time and resources you need to heal.

13.13 Balancing Online and Offline Interactions

In today's digital age, many relationships begin or primarily exist online—through social media, forums, or messaging apps. While these platforms can broaden your horizons, an overreliance on virtual communication can have drawbacks, too. Strive for balance:

- **Positives of Online Socializing**:
    1. **Wider Access**: Meet people from different cultures or with specialized interests that might not be available locally.
    2. **Flexible Interaction**: You can connect on your schedule, which is helpful for busy lifestyles.
- **Possible Pitfalls**:
    1. **Superficial Connections**: It is easy to keep chats shallow if you never meet face-to-face.
    2. **Online Harassment**: The internet can bring negativity or trolls. Knowing how to block or report problematic behavior is essential.
- **Suggestions for Balance**:
    1. **Be Selective**: Follow or connect with accounts that genuinely enrich your life, not those that incite envy or negativity.
    2. **Transition to Offline**: If you form a meaningful online bond and logistics allow, consider meeting in person for deeper connection.
    3. **Limit Screen Time**: Spending too many hours scrolling can leave you feeling disconnected from real-life experiences.

Aim to make technology serve your relationship goals, not overshadow genuine human interactions.

13.14 Cultural Differences and Communication Styles

In a world that is increasingly diverse, you might form relationships with people from different cultural backgrounds. Communication styles, traditions, and expectations can vary widely. To navigate these differences:

- **Learn Actively**: Show interest in another person's culture by asking respectful questions or trying their customs.
- **Stay Open-Minded**: Avoid judging something as "weird" or "wrong" just because it is unfamiliar.
- **Clarify Meanings**: Words or gestures can have different connotations across cultures. When in doubt, politely ask for clarification.
- **Adapt if Needed**: Sometimes you must adjust your approach to connect better. For instance, in some cultures, direct eye contact is a sign of respect, while in others, it might be seen as aggression.

By practicing cultural sensitivity, you expand your social circle and enjoy a richer tapestry of interpersonal experiences.

13.15 The Power of Group Support

Humans have always formed communities, whether for survival or social enrichment. Group support can come in many forms:

1. **Support Groups**: People facing a common challenge—like grief, addiction recovery, or health issues—meet to share stories and coping strategies.
2. **Professional Circles**: Industry-specific associations or networking groups help members exchange knowledge and opportunities.
3. **Recreational Clubs**: Book clubs, sports teams, or crafting circles provide structured ways to bond over shared interests.
4. **Online Forums**: Virtual communities connect individuals from across the globe, offering 24/7 interaction.

The sense of belonging you get from group involvement can significantly reduce feelings of isolation. You also benefit from collective wisdom, as members often share unique insights from their own backgrounds.

13.16 Practical Tips for Supporting Someone in Crisis

Sometimes, a friend or family member needs more support than usual due to a major life event—loss of a job, serious illness, divorce, or the death of a loved one. Offering help compassionately can make a real difference:

1. **Listen Without Judgment**
   - **Safe Space**: Encourage them to share feelings openly. Resist giving quick fixes; often, simply being heard is therapeutic.
2. **Offer Specific Help**
   - **Examples**: Instead of saying "Let me know if you need anything," propose something concrete like bringing a meal, driving them to appointments, or babysitting.
3. **Be Patient**
   - **Recovery or Grief is Not Linear**: They might have ups and downs. Continue checking in, but give them space if they seem to need it.
4. **Respect Their Autonomy**
   - **Avoid Overstepping**: Some people prefer to handle certain tasks alone. Ask before you intervene in their personal affairs.
5. **Encourage Professional Help**
   - **Specialized Support**: If you sense their distress is overwhelming or persistent, gently suggest speaking to a counselor or joining a support group.

By approaching a crisis with sensitivity and understanding, you strengthen your bond and help them see that caring support is available.

13.17 Mending Bridges: When to Reconnect

Not all broken ties are meant to be severed forever. There could be times when you consider rebuilding a strained friendship or familial bond. Here are some factors to consider:

- **Was the Split Toxic or Temporary?** *If serious harm or abuse occurred, reconnecting might not be wise without significant evidence of change.*

If the falling-out was due to a misunderstanding, you might try reconciling.
- **Are Both Parties Willing?** Rebuilding a bond requires effort from both sides. If the other person is uninterested or continues hurtful behaviors, it may be best to let go.
- **Define New Boundaries**: If you do reconnect, be clear about what you can and cannot accept. For instance, limit topics if previous arguments focused on sensitive issues.
- **Move Forward, Not Backward**: Dwelling on old resentments can derail progress. Focus on rebuilding trust in the present if both parties genuinely aim for a healthier dynamic.

Reconciliation can bring renewed support and closure, but only if the relationship is capable of healthy growth moving forward.

13.18 Real-Life Example: Carla's Circle of Support

Carla moved to a new city for a job opportunity. Initially, she felt isolated. Determined to break out of loneliness, she:

- **Joined a Local Hiking Club**: She loved nature, so this step helped her meet others with similar interests. Slowly, she found people to grab coffee with after weekend hikes.
- **Attended Professional Meetups**: Carla also participated in monthly meetups for women in her industry. There, she discovered a mentor who guided her career path.
- **Kept In Touch with Old Friends**: Regular video calls with her childhood friend gave her familiarity and comfort while adjusting to city life.
- **Practiced Setting Boundaries**: At work, Carla gently distanced herself from a coworker who often gossiped, realizing that negative energy did not support her well-being.

Within a year, Carla built a solid support network, blending new and old connections. She felt more grounded, confident, and open to tackling challenges at her job. Her journey demonstrates that proactive steps and mindful choices can create a strong circle of relationships, even in unfamiliar territory.

13.19 Strengthening Community Ties

Beyond one-on-one relationships, engaging with your broader community can offer deep fulfillment. Community ties can be found in neighborhoods, faith groups, cultural organizations, or local initiatives:

- **Attend Local Events**: Fairs, cultural festivals, or neighborhood gatherings can help you meet diverse people in a relaxed setting.
- **Volunteer Locally**: Contributing your time to causes that resonate with you fosters a sense of purpose and introduces you to others who share your passion.
- **Organize Gatherings**: Hosting a small potluck or block party can bring neighbors together, forging new friendships and community spirit.
- **Support Local Businesses**: Frequenting local shops or cafes builds relationships with business owners and fellow patrons over time.

Community involvement can shift your perspective from individual concerns to shared goals, reminding you of the powerful impact people have when they unite.

CHAPTER 14

Overcoming Common Obstacles

14.1 Introduction: Life's Roadblocks Are Inevitable

No matter how skilled, confident, or prepared you are, obstacles will appear in your path. They can come in many forms—financial hurdles, health issues, time constraints, or even unexpected family duties. Instead of viewing these challenges as proof of inadequacy, it is more helpful to see them as normal parts of life that everyone faces. The key difference lies in how you respond.

In this chapter, we will discuss common barriers that women encounter and outline strategic, straightforward ways to handle them. By learning to see obstacles as opportunities for growth, you can stay motivated and move closer to your goals with resilience. Remember, having setbacks or difficulties does not make you a failure; it simply makes you human. With the right mindset and tools, every challenge can become a stepping stone rather than a stumbling block.

14.2 Identifying the Obstacles Holding You Back

The first step in overcoming any obstacle is to define it clearly. Vague worries—like "I'm too busy" or "I don't have enough money"—can feel overwhelming. Pinpointing the exact nature of the challenge helps you find workable solutions. Below are some categories of common obstacles:

1. **Time Management Problems**
   - **Examples**: Procrastinating, juggling multiple roles, spending hours on distractions.
   - **Impact**: You never seem to have enough time for important tasks, leading to stress and missed opportunities.
2. **Financial Struggles**
   - **Examples**: Debt, low income, unexpected medical bills, inadequate savings.

- **Impact**: Monetary stress can limit your ability to invest in education, hobbies, or life goals, affecting confidence and mental health.
3. **Emotional Roadblocks**
    - **Examples**: Fear of failure, chronic self-doubt, or anxiety about the future.
    - **Impact**: You might hesitate to try new things or set ambitious goals due to internal negative voices.
4. **Health Issues**
    - **Examples**: Chronic illness, limited mobility, or mental health challenges like depression.
    - **Impact**: Physical or mental struggles can sap your energy, lower motivation, and require resources such as time and money for treatment.
5. **Lack of Support**
    - **Examples**: Unsupportive family, absent friends, or a negative social environment.
    - **Impact**: Without help or encouragement, tasks feel more daunting, and isolation can damage self-confidence.

Recognizing which category your obstacles fall under—or if they span multiple categories—lets you tackle them with targeted strategies.

14.3 Time Constraints and Procrastination

One of the most common roadblocks is feeling like there are not enough hours in the day. This often goes hand in hand with procrastination. Together, they create a cycle: you feel stressed about limited time, which makes you delay tasks, and as tasks pile up, stress increases. To break this cycle:

1. **Set Clear Priorities**
    - **Simplify**: Decide which projects, errands, or commitments truly matter. Let go of tasks that do not align with your goals or values.
    - **Chunk Tasks**: Break big assignments into small parts. Completing tiny steps can boost motivation to keep going.
2. **Use Time-Blocking**

- **How It Works**: Divide your day into blocks dedicated to specific tasks. For example, use one hour for emails, another for creative work, etc.
- **Benefit**: This structure prevents you from constantly switching tasks, which wastes mental energy.

3. **Address Procrastination Head-On**
   - **Identify Triggers**: Observe when you are most likely to avoid work. Is it when the task seems too complex or boring?
   - **Start Small**: Commit to just five minutes of that dreaded task. Often, once you begin, you find it easier to continue.
   - **Reward Yourself**: After finishing a time block or major chunk, take a short break or enjoy a small treat. Positive reinforcement makes consistency likelier.
4. **Stay Flexible**
   - **Life Happens**: Unexpected events can disrupt your schedule. Rather than beating yourself up, quickly adapt and reschedule tasks as needed.
   - **Routine Updates**: Periodically review your time plan. If something is not working, adjust it instead of giving up.

Effective time management can free you from the last-minute rush, lowering stress and giving you space to focus on what really matters.

14.4 Financial Obstacles and Budgeting Tips

Money worries can be overwhelming. They often lead to feeling trapped or powerless. However, even small steps toward better financial health can make a big difference:

1. **Create a Realistic Budget**
   - **Track Income and Expenses**: Write down all your monthly earnings and expenses. This clarity shows where changes are possible.
   - **Prioritize Necessities**: Rent, utilities, and groceries come first. Reduce optional expenses if you are short on funds.
2. **Build an Emergency Fund**

- **Start Small**: Saving even $10 or $20 per week can add up. Put this into a separate account you are not tempted to use for everyday spending.
- **Automate Saving**: If possible, set up an automatic transfer so you never forget to save.

3. **Deal with Debt Strategically**
   - **High-Interest First**: Pay off debts with the highest interest rates, like credit card balances. Focus extra money on these debts while making minimum payments on others.
   - **Seek Guidance**: If debt is overwhelming, consult a credit counselor or look into reputable debt-management programs.

4. **Increase Income if Possible**
   - **Side Hustles**: If you can, use a skill or hobby for extra income—like freelancing, tutoring, or selling homemade goods.
   - **Ask for a Raise**: If you have been performing well at your job, gather evidence of your achievements and negotiate a pay increase.

5. **Stay Informed**
   - **Financial Education**: Read basic finance books or follow reputable finance blogs. Understanding terms like interest rates, mutual funds, or retirement accounts helps you make wiser decisions.

Overcoming financial obstacles is rarely instant, but consistent efforts can improve your situation over time. Feeling more in control of your finances often boosts overall confidence.

14.5 Emotional Barriers: Fear and Self-Doubt

Emotional roadblocks like anxiety, fear of rejection, or imposter syndrome can halt progress. You might have a great plan yet hold yourself back due to inner voices saying "You can't do this" or "You'll fail." Consider these approaches:

1. **Challenge Negative Thoughts**
   - **Write Them Down**: If you think, "I'm not smart enough," put it on paper and ask, "Is this actually true?"

- **Search for Counter-Evidence**: Reflect on past achievements or times you overcame difficulties—those moments prove you have capabilities.
2. **Practice Visualization**
    - **Positive Outcome**: Close your eyes and imagine succeeding in your goal—completing a presentation, finishing a course, or impressing a client.
    - **Emotional Boost**: This mental rehearsal can reduce stress and make you more comfortable taking real action.
3. **Use Affirmations**
    - **Short Phrases**: Statements like "I am capable" or "I learn from mistakes" can replace self-critical thoughts.
    - **Consistency**: Repeat them daily, ideally out loud or in writing, to reshape your internal dialogue over time.
4. **Seek Support**
    - **Therapy or Coaching**: Mental health professionals can offer tools to manage anxiety or deep-seated fears.
    - **Personal Tribe**: Share your concerns with a friend or mentor who can remind you of your strengths.
5. **Take Incremental Risks**
    - **Stretch Comfort Zones**: Tackle small challenges first, such as speaking up in a meeting or enrolling in a short course.
    - **Learn from Each Step**: Each mini-success can build the confidence to try bigger leaps later.

Overcoming emotional barriers is a gradual process. Consistent, gentle effort can help you believe in yourself, even if part of you remains uncertain.

14.6 Health-Related Setbacks

Physical health challenges—like chronic pain, recurring illnesses, or limited mobility—can significantly slow your progress. Mental health issues—such as depression, anxiety, or PTSD—can also reduce energy and motivation. Here is how to cope:

1. **Seek Professional Help**

- **Medical Team**: Regular check-ups, following treatment plans, and taking prescribed medications can stabilize chronic conditions.
- **Mental Health Therapy**: Therapies like cognitive-behavioral therapy or counseling can teach coping skills for mood disorders or anxiety.

2. **Adjust Goals as Needed**
   - **Realistic Timelines**: Accept that you may need more rest or recovery days than someone without health issues.
   - **Adapt Workflows**: If you have trouble standing, find seated or low-impact exercises. If you experience mental fatigue, schedule tasks in shorter blocks.

3. **Focus on Nutrition and Sleep**
   - **Balanced Diet**: Nutritious meals can strengthen your body's resilience, giving you more energy for daily life.
   - **Ample Rest**: Poor sleep worsens many health conditions. Aim for a calm bedtime routine and limit screen time before bed.

4. **Community Resources**
   - **Support Groups**: Others with similar health issues can share tips, from managing flare-ups to accessing local medical resources.
   - **Accessible Tools**: Use assistive technology or other aids. For instance, speech-to-text software if typing is painful.

5. **Celebrate Small Improvements**
   - **Patience is Key**: Health recovery or management might be slow. Acknowledge progress—even if it is modest.

Prioritizing your well-being does not mean giving up on aspirations. With the right approach, you can still achieve meaningful goals while respecting your body's needs.

14.7 Lack of Social or Emotional Support

Trying to reach milestones alone can be discouraging, especially when you crave a cheerleader or a partner for accountability. If your immediate circle does not provide much support:

1. **Broaden Your Network**

- **Local Groups**: Join community or interest-based clubs, so you are more likely to meet supportive peers.
- **Online Forums**: Look for digital spaces that share your goals, such as healthy living communities or professional forums.

2. **Ask for Specific Help**
   - **Concrete Requests**: Instead of hoping someone will notice your struggle, directly ask a friend, "Could you check in with me once a week to see how I'm doing with my project?"
   - **Exchange Support**: Offer your assistance in return, creating a reciprocal relationship.

3. **Seek Mentors or Allies**
   - **Professional Fields**: If you are building a career, try to connect with someone in your industry who can guide you.
   - **Volunteer or Community Circles**: Places where people bond over shared values can lead to lasting friendships.

4. **Rely on Self-Encouragement Temporarily**
   - **Journaling**: Record achievements and lessons learned, acting as your own cheerleader.
   - **Positive Reminders**: Place notes around your home with inspiring quotes or reminders of why your goal matters.

While external support is wonderful, you can still move forward even when it is lacking. Over time, new connections or changing life circumstances might bring stronger support your way.

14.8 Fear of Failure and Perfectionism

Sometimes, the biggest obstacle is the unrelenting desire to do everything flawlessly. This fear of making mistakes can paralyze action, as you wait for the "perfect" time or condition. To break free:

1. **Redefine Failure**
   - **Learning Experience**: View mistakes as data points. They show what works and what does not, helping you adjust more intelligently.
   - **Progress Over Perfection**: Celebrate partial successes, improvements, or attempts. Doing something at 80% quality might be more beneficial than not doing it at all.

2. **Set Flexible Goals**
   - **Include "Testing" Phases**: Instead of planning everything in detail at once, allow room to test ideas and pivot if necessary.
   - **Break Perfection**: Occasionally, intentionally do a task less than perfectly to train yourself to cope with imperfection—like making a simple, slightly messy meal instead of an elaborate dish.
3. **Gather Feedback**
   - **Constructive Insights**: Asking others for input can help you see which aspects need refining versus which are already good enough.
   - **Balanced Perspective**: Realizing you do some things well can counterbalance your focus on flaws.
4. **Try New Things Regularly**
   - **Small Risks**: Sign up for a new class, speak up in a group discussion, or experiment with a creative hobby.
   - **Build Resilience**: The more you face challenges, the more you train yourself to adapt and improve, not freeze in fear.

A life lived in fear of failure often leads to missed opportunities. Embracing imperfection and seeing failure as part of growth can release you from the chains of perfectionism.

14.9 Time of Transition: Managing Life Shifts

Life transitions—like moving to a new city, changing careers, or entering a new relationship—can spark doubt and confusion. During transitional phases:

1. **Acknowledge Emotional Turmoil**
   - **Stress is Normal**: Recognize that transitions inherently carry uncertainty. Feeling anxious does not mean you made the wrong decision.
   - **Give Yourself Grace**: Avoid criticizing yourself for not adjusting instantly.
2. **Plan, but Stay Flexible**
   - **Broad Outline**: Create a step-by-step approach if you are switching careers—like updating your resume, networking, taking relevant courses.

        - **Wiggle Room**: Accept that not everything will go as planned. Build slack into your schedule for learning curves.
3. **Draw on Past Transitions**
     - **Reflect**: Recall earlier times you faced big changes, such as starting college or recovering from a major challenge. What helped you get through those periods?
     - **Apply Lessons**: Use successful strategies from the past—like journaling, seeking a mentor, or focusing on short-term achievable goals.
4. **Self-Care Reminders**
     - **Physical Health**: Exercise, balanced meals, and enough sleep boost your ability to handle stress.
     - **Mental Breaks**: Schedule small pockets of relaxation—listening to music, reading for fun, or taking walks—so your mind can recharge.

Transitions can become transformative experiences if approached with patience and openness to learning.

14.10 External Pressures and Societal Expectations

Many women face external pressures about how they should look, behave, or progress in life—often intensifying feelings of inadequacy. Coping with these demands requires:

1. **Clarify Your Own Values**
     - **Self-Check**: Ask, "Whose standard am I trying to meet?" and "Do I genuinely care about this, or am I seeking approval?"
     - **Redirect Focus**: Spend energy on goals that resonate with your principles, rather than external validation.
2. **Seek Diverse Role Models**
     - **Representation Matters**: Follow stories or social media accounts of women who break stereotypes, showing multiple ways to be successful or happy.
     - **Challenge Narrow Norms**: Acknowledge that there is no one "correct" life path. Everyone's journey looks different.
3. **Practice Assertiveness**

- **Set Boundaries**: If relatives or acquaintances press you on personal matters—like marriage or having kids—firmly but politely state that you are content with your timeline.
- **External Criticism**: When someone pushes you to conform, calmly express your stance. You do not have to explain every detail, only that you have chosen differently.

4. **Cultivate Inner Validation**
   - **Internal Scorecard**: Measure success by whether you feel aligned with your values and personal growth, not by society's shifting standards.
   - **Celebrate Unique Paths**: Remind yourself that "fitting in" is less important than living authentically.

By defining your life on your own terms, societal pressures gradually lose their grip, giving you room to flourish on your chosen path.

14.11 Overcoming Obstacles in Education or Career Growth

Whether you are pursuing higher education, aiming for a promotion, or switching careers, obstacles often arise. Common ones include lacking qualifications, balancing family duties, or facing workplace discrimination. Here are strategies:

1. **Skills Assessment**
   - **Identify Gaps**: Determine which skills or qualifications you need, and research how to obtain them—be it through online courses, workshops, or certifications.
   - **Leverage Current Strengths**: Market or highlight your transferable skills, such as teamwork, problem-solving, or communication.
2. **Find Allies at Work or School**
   - **Study Groups or Peer Partners**: Collaborative learning can alleviate struggles in tough subjects.
   - **Coworker Connections**: Networking internally can open doors to mentorship or new roles.
3. **Tackle Discrimination or Bias**
   - **Document Incidents**: If you face unfair treatment, keep records of events.

- ○ **Seek Guidance**: Consult HR, a union representative, or a trusted mentor about possible actions.
- ○ **Mentally Separate Self-Worth**: Remember, bias is a reflection of others' prejudices, not your competence or value.

4. **Manage Family Commitments**
   - ○ **Scheduling**: If you have caregiving responsibilities, coordinate with family members or friends to create study or work blocks.
   - ○ **Online and Flexible Programs**: Many educational institutions or workplaces now offer part-time, remote, or evening options to accommodate busy schedules.

Education and career progress do not always follow a straight line. Adapting to obstacles with a proactive mindset can ultimately deepen your professional credibility and personal growth.

14.12 Tools for Accountability and Progress Tracking

Accountability can significantly help in battling common obstacles. Here's how:

1. **Goal-Setting Apps**
   - ○ **Features**: Some apps let you break down big projects, set deadlines, and send reminders.
   - ○ **Motivation**: Watching digital progress bars fill up can be surprisingly satisfying.
2. **Accountability Partner**
   - ○ **Mutual Check-Ins**: Meet or message weekly, discussing each other's progress, setbacks, and next steps.
   - ○ **Problem-Solving Buddy**: Brainstorm solutions for each other when stuck.
3. **Visual Reminders**
   - ○ **Bulletin Board**: Place a calendar or list of goals somewhere visible at home or in your office.
   - ○ **Sticky Notes**: Jot down positive messages or small tasks and keep them on your desk or mirror.
4. **Regular Self-Evaluations**
   - ○ **Weekly Reflection**: Spend 10 minutes each weekend asking, "What went well? What can I improve?"

- **Adjust Goals**: If a method is not working, try a different strategy rather than abandoning your objective.

By systematically tracking your efforts, you maintain focus, celebrate incremental wins, and catch problems early before they derail your progress.

14.13 Learning from Setbacks

No matter how well you plan, sometimes you will stumble—maybe a product launch fails, a job application is rejected, or you face an unexpected personal emergency. Responding effectively is key:

1. **Acceptance**
   - **Feel the Emotions**: Anger, sadness, or disappointment are normal. Recognize them without judgment.
   - **Avoid Dwelling on "What Ifs"**: Replay key moments only to extract lessons, not to torment yourself.
2. **Lesson Extraction**
   - **Specific Questions**: Ask, "Which part could I have done differently? Was the timing off, or did I lack certain resources?"
   - **Document**: Write down insights in a journal. Future you can benefit from this reflection.
3. **Plan Revisions**
   - **Tweak the Approach**: If a marketing campaign did not work, find a new angle or audience. If a study method failed, explore alternative learning techniques.
   - **Seek Expert Advice**: Talk to someone who has experienced similar setbacks for fresh perspectives.
4. **Rebuild Confidence**
   - **List Past Successes**: Reflect on times you overcame difficulties before—this reaffirms your resilience.
   - **Small Next Step**: Even if you are discouraged, performing one positive action can rekindle motivation, like updating your resume or signing up for a new course.

Turning setbacks into growth opportunities fosters a mindset where no challenge is insurmountable; each merely represents another chance to learn and adapt.

14.14 Real-Life Example: Sharon's Determination

Sharon had always dreamed of opening a small bakery. She loved baking pastries for family events and felt confident in her skills. However, obstacles loomed: she had a limited budget, minimal business experience, and a full-time job. At first, Sharon felt overwhelmed, questioning whether her dream was realistic.

Undeterred, she broke down her goals:

- **Financial Planning**: Sharon learned budgeting by reading articles and talking to a friend who worked in finance. She saved a portion of each paycheck, cutting back on non-essentials like eating out.
- **Finding Time**: Sharon dedicated weekends to developing her recipes and practicing new baking techniques. Instead of watching TV, she used early mornings for market research.
- **Seeking Support**: She joined an online bakers' forum and received guidance from experienced professionals, forging valuable friendships.
- **Starting Small**: Rather than leasing a storefront immediately, Sharon tested her menu by selling pastries at local farmers' markets. Her products sold well, generating enough income to reinvest.
- **Adapting After Flops**: When her initial fancy cupcake designs did not sell, she polled customers to see what they preferred. She switched to simpler, more classic flavors, which quickly became a hit.

Little by little, Sharon's plan fell into place. Within two years, she transitioned to part-time work and then opened a modest bakery booth. Eventually, her consistent approach led her to a permanent bakery space. Despite countless setbacks—including machinery breakdowns and tough competition—Sharon's methodical handling of obstacles kept her dream alive.

14.15 Developing a Resourceful Mindset

A resourceful mindset encourages you to see problems not as dead ends but as puzzles. You seek alternatives, gather information, and harness creativity. Strengthen resourcefulness by:

1. **Asking "How?" Instead of "Why Me?"**
   - **Solution-Oriented**: Instead of lamenting a problem's existence, brainstorm ways to fix, minimize, or circumvent it.
2. **Building Knowledge**
   - **Read and Research**: Inform yourself about subjects related to your goals or challenges.
   - **Ask Experts**: Reach out politely to people who have the expertise or experiences you lack.
3. **Embrace Creativity**
   - **Alternative Approaches**: If plan A fails, consider plan B, C, or D. Is there an unconventional path that might work?
   - **Trial and Error**: Test solutions in small ways. If something does not work, refine it rather than discarding the entire idea.
4. **Networking**
   - **Collaborations**: Sometimes working with a partner—who has complementary skills—can help you tackle complex problems more effectively.
   - **Information Exchange**: Offer your skills in return. Trading favors or knowledge can open new doors.

Resourcefulness transforms obstacles into challenges that spark your creativity and willingness to learn. This mental shift can make any problem feel surmountable.

14.16 Healthy Coping Mechanisms During High Stress

When multiple obstacles converge or a particularly big one arises, stress can skyrocket. Use healthy coping tools to maintain equilibrium:

1. **Mindful Breaks**
   - **Deep Breathing**: Spend one minute inhaling and exhaling slowly, focusing on each breath.
   - **Nature Escapes**: If possible, take short walks in a park or by water to clear your head.
2. **Physical Outlets**
   - **Exercise**: Even 15 minutes of stretching or a brisk walk can release tension.
   - **Relaxation Techniques**: Activities like yoga, progressive muscle relaxation, or gentle dancing.

3. **Emotional Expression**
   - **Journaling**: Write freely about your feelings without judgment. This can unburden your mind.
   - **Artistic Endeavors**: Painting, knitting, or playing an instrument can soothe anxiety.
4. **Professional Support**
   - **Therapy**: A counselor can help you navigate intense stress.
   - **Support Lines**: Many communities offer helplines for people in crisis or simply needing to talk.

These techniques create pockets of calm in a stormy period, preventing burnout and enabling you to tackle obstacles with a clearer mind.

14.17 Learning When to Let Go or Pivot

Sometimes, the smartest move is to modify or leave a goal behind. Clinging to a path that no longer aligns with your values or that demands an unrealistic toll on your health can become counterproductive. Consider:

1. **Signs It May Be Time to Pivot**
   - **Consistent Burnout**: Despite repeated attempts to balance your schedule, you remain chronically exhausted.
   - **Shifting Priorities**: Your life context changed—maybe you discovered a new passion or faced new family responsibilities.
   - **Ongoing Conflict**: If you constantly fight with key stakeholders—like a toxic business partner or an unyielding manager—it might be time for a different environment.
2. **Self-Reflection**
   - **Ask Why**: Is your desire to continue based on genuine passion, or is it driven by not wanting to appear like a quitter?
   - **Pros and Cons**: Objectively evaluate the benefits of pushing forward versus trying a new route.
3. **Exit Strategies**
   - **Gradual Transition**: If leaving a job or major commitment, plan financially and emotionally so the shift is smooth.
   - **Closure**: Communicate your decision to relevant parties respectfully. Let them know you are stepping away for well-considered reasons.

Letting go of a goal that no longer serves you is not failure. It can free you to pursue endeavors that better match your evolving situation or spark genuine excitement.

14.18 Practical Steps for Turning Obstacles into Action Plans

Once you identify an obstacle, craft an action plan to address it. Here is a simple structure:

1. **Define the Obstacle Clearly**
    - **Example**: "I want to return to college, but I cannot afford tuition."
2. **Brainstorm Possible Solutions**
    - **Quantity Over Quality**: List all ideas, even if some seem impractical at first (scholarships, part-time jobs, negotiating tuition, online courses, etc.).
3. **Evaluate Feasibility**
    - **Narrow Down**: From the list, pick the top two or three most viable options. Consider time, financial realities, and personal strengths.
4. **Create Actionable Steps**
    - **Be Specific**: "Research 5 scholarship programs by next Friday," "Talk to a financial advisor at the college within two weeks."
5. **Set a Timeline**
    - **Short-Term Goals**: Weekly or monthly tasks that show progress.
    - **Long-Term Milestones**: Where you want to be in 6 months, 1 year, etc.
6. **Check Progress Regularly**
    - **Adjust if Needed**: If a chosen solution proves too costly or time-consuming, pivot to another idea.

Turning each roadblock into a structured plan can prevent feelings of helplessness. You regain a sense of control and direction.

CHAPTER 15

The Role of Spirituality or Mindfulness

15.1 Introduction: Finding Inner Peace and Purpose

Many people think spirituality and mindfulness are only for religious communities or people who meditate daily on a mountain. In reality, spirituality and mindfulness can be everyday practices that help you stay calm, centered, and in touch with what truly matters. For women, in particular, life can become extremely busy, with responsibilities tugging in different directions. Amid all this, spirituality or mindfulness can serve as an anchor—a gentle reminder that there is more to life than tasks, deadlines, or the opinions of others.

In this chapter, we will explore what spirituality and mindfulness mean in simple terms. We will look at how they can benefit your mental health, relationships, and personal growth. Whether you follow a specific faith, consider yourself spiritual without religion, or simply want to be more present in each moment, these concepts can enrich your life. By learning practical ways to include mindfulness or spirituality in your daily routine, you can feel more grounded and at peace, even during hectic times.

15.2 Understanding Spirituality Beyond Religion

Spirituality can be a tricky word because different people define it differently. Some see it as connected to a specific religious belief, like attending a church, mosque, temple, or synagogue. Others experience spirituality in nature, art, or simply a sense of awe at the beauty of the universe. In a broader sense, spirituality often involves:

1. **A Sense of Connection**
   - Feeling that you are part of something bigger, whether that is a community, nature, or a universal force.

- Recognizing that your life has meaning beyond day-to-day tasks or immediate goals.
2. **Inner Reflection**
    - Taking time to explore your deepest thoughts and emotions, asking questions like, "What is my purpose?" or "How do I want to treat others?"
3. **Values and Ethics**
    - Spirituality can guide you to live in alignment with principles such as compassion, honesty, or kindness, regardless of your religious affiliation.
4. **Personal Growth**
    - Many spiritual paths encourage self-improvement, forgiveness, and living with humility or gratitude.

You can be spiritual without belonging to a formal religion, or you can be religious and spiritual at the same time. The important thing is finding what resonates with you personally, helping you feel more fulfilled and connected to the world around you.

15.3 Defining Mindfulness in Daily Life

Mindfulness is the practice of paying full attention to the present moment. Instead of letting your thoughts drift to the future or past, you focus on the "now." This does not mean ignoring your responsibilities, but rather learning to notice what you are doing and feeling in real time. Key aspects of mindfulness include:

1. **Nonjudgmental Awareness**
    - Observing your thoughts, emotions, or surroundings without labeling them as "good" or "bad."
    - Accepting whatever arises, whether it is a pleasant feeling like joy or an uncomfortable emotion like anxiety.
2. **Intentional Focus**
    - Choosing one thing at a time to pay attention to—such as your breath, a task, or a conversation.
    - Letting go of distractions or mental chatter by gently redirecting your mind whenever it drifts.
3. **Being Present**

- Fully experiencing each moment—tasting your food instead of eating hurriedly or truly listening to a friend instead of planning your response.
- Noticing small details, like the texture of an orange peel or the sound of leaves rustling.

4. **Self-Compassion**
   - In mindfulness, you treat yourself with kindness when your mind wanders or you feel overwhelmed.
   - You learn to gently bring yourself back to the present without frustration or blame.

Mindfulness can be practiced anytime—while eating, walking, washing dishes, or even during a stressful meeting. By grounding yourself in the now, you often reduce anxiety and become more in tune with your true needs and feelings.

15.4 How Spirituality and Mindfulness Boost Confidence

You might wonder how these two concepts link to feeling more confident. The answer lies in what happens when you cultivate a calmer, more centered mind:

1. **Inner Stability**
   - When life's storms hit—like losing a job or facing criticism—spiritual or mindful practices can help you remain steady rather than panic.
   - You trust that you can handle challenges because you have anchored yourself in a deeper sense of purpose or calm.
2. **Clarity of Values**
   - Spiritual reflection often clarifies what is truly important to you—such as kindness or integrity. Knowing your values can guide your decisions and boost self-assurance because you act in line with who you are.
3. **Reduced Negative Self-Talk**
   - Mindfulness helps you notice harsh, automatic thoughts like "I'm a failure" or "I can't do this." By simply observing these thoughts, you learn they are not absolute truths.
   - Over time, this makes you less likely to be consumed by negativity, thus increasing self-esteem.

4. **Resilience**
    - Spiritual teachings, such as forgiveness, humility, and gratitude, can strengthen your ability to bounce back from setbacks.
    - Rather than feeling crushed by difficulties, you may view them as part of life's journey, which in turn keeps your confidence intact.
5. **Deeper Self-Awareness**
    - By sitting quietly in meditation or prayer, you get to know yourself more deeply—your strengths, fears, and hopes. Self-awareness is a powerful foundation for genuine self-confidence.

15.5 Practical Ways to Cultivate Mindfulness

Building mindfulness does not require drastic lifestyle changes. Small daily habits can lead to significant benefits over time. Here are simple approaches:

1. **Mindful Breathing**
    - **How**: Spend a minute focusing on your breath. Inhale slowly, then exhale gently. Notice how your abdomen moves.
    - **When**: Do this first thing in the morning, during a work break, or before bed.
2. **Body Scan**
    - **How**: Close your eyes and mentally scan your body from head to toe. Observe where you feel tension or ease.
    - **Benefit**: This reduces physical stress and promotes relaxation.
3. **Mindful Eating**
    - **How**: Take small bites, chew slowly, and notice the flavors, textures, and aromas of your food.
    - **Why**: This prevents you from rushing meals and helps you enjoy what you eat, often leading to healthier eating habits.
4. **Single-Tasking**
    - **How**: Instead of multitasking, focus on one job at a time—like washing dishes without also scrolling through your phone.
    - **Result**: You complete tasks more efficiently and with less stress, feeling more in control.
5. **Mindful Walking**

- **How**: Walk at a normal pace but pay attention to your steps, the ground under your feet, and your surroundings. Notice the breeze or sunlight.
- **Gain**: Combines movement with meditation, grounding you in the present.

These small exercises can be interwoven into your regular day. Even five minutes of mindful practice can calm your mind and enhance your awareness.

15.6 Different Approaches to Spiritual Practice

If you feel drawn to explore spirituality, there is no one-size-fits-all method. The path you choose can be deeply personal:

1. **Religious Path**
   - **Commitment**: Attending services, reading sacred texts, or practicing religious rituals can provide structure and community support.
   - **Guidance**: Religious traditions often have leaders—priests, rabbis, imams, or monks—who can offer teachings and help with spiritual questions.
2. **Nature-Based Spirituality**
   - **Connection**: Spending time outdoors, observing the changing seasons, or tending to a garden can foster awe and gratitude.
   - **Rituals**: Some people find meaning in marking solstices or equinoxes, reflecting on the harmony of the natural world.
3. **Personal Reflection**
   - **Journaling**: Writing down your thoughts, prayers, or questions can turn into a sacred practice, revealing deeper insights about your worries or dreams.
   - **Meditation**: Sitting quietly with the intention to sense a higher power or universal love can nurture inner peace and compassion.
4. **Creative Expression**
   - **Art and Music**: Painting, dancing, or playing an instrument with full presence can feel like a spiritual experience, connecting you to something beyond ordinary concerns.

- **Gratitude Lists**: Listing things you are thankful for daily can spark a sense of wonder and appreciation.
5. **Service to Others**
    - **Volunteering**: Helping people in need or participating in community projects can be a spiritual act, reminding you of the shared humanity that binds us.
    - **Acts of Kindness**: Even small gestures—like supporting a friend or smiling at a stranger—can feed your spiritual sense of empathy and unity.

Each path has its own flavor, but the core idea is to find a practice that inspires you, aligns with your values, and helps you grow.

15.7 Overcoming Obstacles to Spiritual or Mindful Practice

Sometimes you might feel that spirituality or mindfulness is too "abstract" or time-consuming. Here are common obstacles and ways around them:

1. **Busy Schedule**
    - **Strategy**: Start small. Even two minutes of deep breathing before bed can be a powerful habit. You do not need an hour of meditation to gain benefits.
    - **Integration**: Combine mindful moments with everyday tasks, like brushing your teeth with full awareness or pausing for a breath when a phone rings.
2. **Skepticism**
    - **Approach**: Understand that mindfulness and spirituality do not require you to believe in anything supernatural if that does not resonate. Think of them as mental and emotional training, like exercise for the mind.
    - **Trial Period**: Test it out for a set number of days or weeks. Observe how it affects your mood or stress level.
3. **Fear of Judgment**
    - **Reality**: Friends or family may not share your newfound interest. They could see it as odd or "unnecessary."
    - **Response**: Practice privately at first, or share only with people who are open-minded. Over time, they might notice positive changes in you and become more accepting.

4. **Mind Wandering**
   - **Normal**: In meditation or prayer, the mind often drifts. That does not mean you are "doing it wrong."
   - **Solution**: Gently bring your focus back each time you notice it wandering. This exercise is the essence of mindfulness—it trains your mental muscles.
5. **Emotional Discomfort**
   - **Why**: Sitting in stillness or reflecting spiritually can bring up old worries or sadness.
   - **Healthy Coping**: If strong emotions surface, acknowledge them and consider seeking professional support if needed (e.g., therapy). This process can eventually lead to healing.

With patience and practical strategies, these obstacles become manageable, allowing you to enjoy the benefits of a spiritual or mindful lifestyle.

15.8 Relationship Between Mindfulness and Stress Management

Many women juggle multiple roles—mother, caregiver, employee, student, community volunteer. This juggling act can be stressful. Mindfulness works as a natural stress reliever:

1. **Cortisol Reduction**
   - **Science**: Regular meditation has been linked to lower cortisol levels (the stress hormone), which helps reduce tension in the body.
   - **Benefit**: You feel calmer and less rushed.
2. **Preventing Overreaction**
   - **Example**: If your child spills juice on your laptop or you receive upsetting news at work, mindfulness can help you pause and breathe before snapping.
   - **Outcome**: Problems get resolved more calmly, and relationships remain smoother.
3. **Emotional Regulation**
   - **Skill**: By noticing emotions as they arise, you become better at managing anger, anxiety, or sadness before they escalate.

- **Result**: Decision-making improves because you respond thoughtfully instead of impulsively.
4. **Better Sleep**
   - **Practice**: A short mindful session before bed—focusing on your breath or using a guided meditation—can calm mental chatter.
   - **Rest**: Good sleep supports overall well-being, giving you more energy to face daily challenges.

When stress is managed effectively, your confidence grows. You trust yourself to handle surprises and remain balanced under pressure.

15.9 How Spiritual Communities Can Support You

Joining a spiritual community—such as a church, meditation group, or spiritual circle—can be a profound source of support:

1. **Shared Purpose**
   - **Connection**: Meeting people with similar beliefs or practices builds instant rapport. You have a common foundation to discuss and explore.
   - **Learning**: You can share experiences, learn from others' journeys, and find mentors who guide you along your spiritual path.
2. **Social Support**
   - **Encouragement**: If you face personal struggles—like job loss or illness—members of a caring community often step in to help or simply listen.
   - **Shared Activities**: Group rituals, retreats, or volunteer events can deepen bonds and provide a sense of belonging.
3. **Moral and Ethical Development**
   - **Discussions**: Many spiritual groups hold talks or study sessions on topics like compassion, forgiveness, or gratitude.
   - **Application**: You get a chance to apply these principles in real life, reinforcing positive behavior and emotional maturity.
4. **Accountability**
   - **Consistency**: Attending weekly gatherings or prayer sessions encourages you to maintain your practice, which can be crucial for building a habit.

- **Friendly Reminder**: Seeing others continue their spiritual work can motivate you to keep going, even when personal life gets hectic.

Of course, not every community is perfect. If you encounter group dynamics that feel rigid, judgmental, or contrary to your values, it is okay to seek another place that suits you better.

15.10 Real-Life Example: Priya's Journey with Mindful Living

Priya was a working mother of two who felt perpetually stressed. Between her full-time job, her children's needs, and household duties, she never paused. She constantly worried about the future—bills, college funds, her aging parents—yet felt too drained to do anything constructive about these concerns.

One day, a friend recommended a short mindfulness course. Although skeptical, Priya gave it a try, initially practicing just five minutes of mindful breathing each evening. She realized how tense her shoulders and jaw were, something she had never paid attention to before. After a couple of weeks, she noticed a slight improvement in her overall mood. Encouraged, Priya began journaling for a few minutes every morning, writing about her worries rather than letting them swirl in her head.

Over months, Priya added brief walking meditations on her lunch break. She also used a simple gratitude practice before bedtime, listing three small things that brought her joy. Gradually, she found herself less reactive. When her kids argued, she paused to take a breath instead of yelling. At work, she tackled projects in focused bursts rather than multitasking. Though life remained busy, Priya reported feeling more in control and "lighter" inside. This shift grew her confidence; she believed that she could handle challenges without unraveling.

Priya did not join a formal religious group, but she embraced spirituality in a personal way—valuing gratitude, presence, and compassion. This approach shaped her family life and career, demonstrating that even small, consistent mindfulness habits can lead to profound change.

15.11 Healing and Forgiveness Through Spiritual Practice

Hurt and resentment can weigh heavily on the heart, damaging self-esteem and overall mental health. Spiritual practices often encourage forgiveness and healing, which in turn free you from emotional burdens:

1. **Understanding Forgiveness**
    - **Myth**: Forgiving does not mean excusing harmful behavior or forgetting the pain caused.
    - **Reality**: It means releasing the intense anger or bitterness so it no longer dominates your thoughts and feelings.
2. **Spiritual Tools for Forgiveness**
    - **Prayer or Meditation**: Many traditions include prayers asking for strength to forgive. Repeating these can soften anger over time.
    - **Imagining Compassion**: Picture the person who hurt you, acknowledging their own struggles. This does not excuse them, but it can reduce your rage.
3. **Self-Forgiveness**
    - **Why It Matters**: We can be harshest on ourselves, replaying mistakes or regrets constantly.
    - **Process**: Offer yourself the same mercy you would a friend. Journaling or quiet reflection can help you see your missteps as part of being human, ripe for growth.
4. **Benefits**
    - **Emotional Release**: Letting go of grudges or self-hatred creates space for healthier emotions, like empathy or acceptance.
    - **Better Relationships**: You approach people with kindness and openness, rather than suspicion or guardedness.

Forgiveness is often a journey, not a one-time event. Yet the process can be deeply liberating, fueling a renewed sense of self-worth and calm.

15.12 Incorporating Mindfulness at Work

If you have a busy job, you may think there is no room for spiritual or mindful practices. However, you can weave them into your workday in practical ways:

1. **Morning Check-In**
   - **Routine**: Arrive a few minutes early, sit at your desk, and take three deep breaths before turning on your computer.
   - **Focus**: Ask yourself, "What do I want to accomplish today, and how do I want to treat my coworkers?"
2. **Mindful Breaks**
   - **Micro-Pauses**: After completing a task, close your eyes for 20 seconds and just breathe.
   - **Lunchtime**: If possible, step outside for a short walk or at least stand near a window, observing the scene mindfully.
3. **Listening Skills**
   - **Meetings**: Practice mindful listening—paying full attention to whoever is speaking rather than rehearsing your reply.
   - **Result**: Reduced misunderstandings and deeper collaboration with colleagues.
4. **End-of-Day Reflection**
   - **Wrap-Up**: Before leaving, think about what went well and what could be improved.
   - **Gratitude**: Acknowledge something positive—a project you finished or help from a coworker.

Such small actions can transform work stress into a more balanced experience, improving both performance and personal well-being.

15.13 Connecting Mindfulness with Creativity

Creativity blossoms when the mind is free from clutter and stress. Mindfulness can unlock your creative potential by:

1. **Opening Space**
   - **Mental Clearance**: By quieting the constant stream of thoughts, you create room for new ideas to surface.
   - **Encouraging Curiosity**: You become more curious about your surroundings and experiences, fueling artistic or inventive thinking.
2. **Non-Judgment**

- **Experimentation**: Mindfulness teaches you not to judge your creations too harshly. This willingness to experiment leads to more original work.
- **Resilience**: If an idea fails, you simply note it and move on, instead of berating yourself.
3. **Focus on Process**
    - **Immersion**: Whether painting, writing, or crafting, being fully present in the act makes it more enjoyable and often yields better outcomes.
    - **Reduced Pressure**: You care less about a perfect end product and more about the learning process.

This link between mindfulness and creativity can apply to cooking, problem-solving, or any pursuit that benefits from fresh perspectives.

15.14 The Science Behind It All

A growing body of research supports the benefits of spirituality and mindfulness:

- **Mindfulness Meditation**: Studies show it can help lower blood pressure, reduce anxiety, and even improve sleep quality.
- **Spiritual Well-Being**: Some research indicates that a sense of spiritual connection correlates with higher optimism, better coping skills, and increased satisfaction in life.
- **Brain Changes**: Regular meditators often display increased gray matter in brain regions linked to memory and emotional regulation.
- **Stress Hormones**: Simple mindfulness exercises can decrease cortisol levels, helping you manage everyday tension more effectively.

Although not a magic cure, these practices offer natural and accessible tools for emotional balance and mental health.

15.15 Common Misconceptions

Some misconceptions might discourage you from exploring spirituality or mindfulness:

1. **"I Must Sit Silently for Hours"**
   - **Reality**: Even brief, 2-5 minute sessions have positive effects. Consistency matters more than long durations.
2. **"It Conflicts with My Religion"**
   - **Reality**: People from diverse religious backgrounds use mindfulness or spiritual reflection, tailoring it to their beliefs.
3. **"I Have to Be Perfectly Calm"**
   - **Reality**: Emotions fluctuate. Spiritual or mindful practice is about noticing emotions, not erasing them.
4. **"It's Too 'Soft' or 'Unproductive'"**
   - **Reality**: Mindfulness can improve focus and productivity by preventing burnout. Spiritual virtues like compassion often lead to stronger connections and a more positive influence on those around you.
5. **"I'm Too Stressed to Sit Still"**
   - **Reality**: That stress is a reason to try it, not a barrier. If sitting is uncomfortable, consider a walking meditation or gentle yoga.

Clearing up these misunderstandings can help you approach spirituality or mindfulness with an open mind and realistic expectations.

15.16 Combining Spirituality with Other Personal Growth Efforts

You have already learned about healthy habits, goal-setting, managing fear, and building better relationships in previous chapters. Spiritual or mindful practices can blend seamlessly with these self-improvement areas:

1. **Goals and Motivation**
   - **Example**: If you are setting weight-loss or career goals, mindfulness helps you stay present during each step—like choosing healthier meals or focusing on work tasks diligently.

2. **Habit Formation**
   - **Bridge**: Combine a new spiritual habit (e.g., short morning meditation) with an existing one (brewing coffee). This anchors spiritual practice into your routine.
3. **Stress and Fear Management**
   - **Reinforcement**: While tools like deep breathing or affirmations help in anxious moments, a spiritual outlook adds a broader perspective that soothes long-term worries.
4. **Relationships**
   - **Impact**: Practicing compassion or forgiveness from a spiritual viewpoint can improve your personal and professional relationships.
5. **Confidence Building**
   - **Underlying Strength**: Feeling connected to something bigger or having mindful awareness can make you more assured in pursuing new opportunities.

By weaving spirituality or mindfulness into other aspects of your personal growth, you create a supportive ecosystem that nurtures overall well-being.

15.17 Handling Skeptical Friends or Family

Not everyone around you will share your interest in spirituality or mindfulness. Some may even mock it. Here is how to handle that gracefully:

1. **Stay Confident**
   - **Your Choice**: Remember, this practice is for your benefit, not anyone else's approval.
   - **Avoid Arguments**: If someone dismisses your activities, calmly acknowledge their viewpoint without getting defensive.
2. **Provide Small Insights**
   - **Mention Benefits**: You could say, "I find it reduces my stress" or "It helps me feel more focused" rather than debating any mystical aspect.
   - **Share Facts**: If they are open, mention scientific research linking mindfulness to better health.
3. **Invite Curiosity, Not Pressure**

- **Optional**: Let them try a short meditation or breathing exercise with you if they show interest.
- **No Coercion**: If they remain uninterested, respect that choice. Everyone has their own path.

Ultimately, your spiritual or mindful journey is personal. Over time, some skeptics may warm up upon seeing positive changes in your demeanor and stress levels.

15.18 Setting Realistic Expectations

Mindfulness and spirituality are not quick fixes. They often bring subtle improvements that grow with consistent practice:

1. **Patience is Key**
   - **Gradual Shifts**: You might notice small changes—like slightly improved patience or easier sleep—before bigger transformations.
   - **Plateaus**: Sometimes you will feel stuck, not experiencing new insights. Persevere; these plateaus are part of any growth journey.
2. **Flexible Approach**
   - **Experiment**: Try different meditation styles or spiritual readings to see what resonates.
   - **Life Changes**: Your spiritual needs may evolve with major life events—like marriage, parenthood, or loss. Adjust your practice accordingly.
3. **No Final Destination**
   - **Continuous Learning**: Mindfulness and spirituality are lifelong paths. There is always more to explore and refine.
   - **Celebrate Mileposts**: Recognize and appreciate each moment of clarity or peace as it comes.

This mindset removes pressure to achieve instant enlightenment or perfect calm. Instead, you appreciate the journey, letting each day be a chance to grow a little more.

15.19 Bringing Mindfulness into Group or Family Life

While much of mindfulness is personal, you can also share it with loved ones:

1. **Family Routine**
    - **Example**: Spend a minute of silence together before meals, allowing everyone to breathe and relax.
    - **Outcome**: This fosters a calmer atmosphere at home and teaches children about patience.
2. **Joint Activities**
    - **Option**: Try a family nature walk where phones are off, and each person notices small details—birds singing, leaves rustling.
    - **Connection**: Such shared moments can increase closeness and mutual understanding.
3. **Partner Meditation**
    - **Practice**: If you have a romantic partner, consider meditating side by side. You do not have to speak; just share a peaceful environment.
    - **Deeper Bond**: This can bring a sense of unity and support, reminding both of you that you are on this life journey together.
4. **Mindful Conflict Resolution**
    - **Technique**: When disagreements arise, each person takes a few mindful breaths before speaking.
    - **Effect**: People tend to respond rather than react, leading to more empathetic communication.

By inviting others, you make spiritual or mindful practices a collective experience, which can multiply the benefits and create a harmonious living environment.

CHAPTER 16

Career and Ambition

16.1 Introduction: Defining Your Own Version of Success

For many women, career paths and personal ambitions form a major part of identity and daily life. You might dream of climbing the corporate ladder, building your own business, pursuing a creative passion, or excelling in a trade or profession. Whatever your goals, the journey is rarely straightforward. There can be roadblocks such as limited opportunities, bias, or juggling family responsibilities. Yet, a well-chosen and well-managed career can bring not only financial stability but also a sense of achievement, confidence, and purpose.

In this chapter, we will explore how to develop a career mindset that is both ambitious and realistic. We will discuss setting clear goals, dealing with workplace challenges, and adapting to changing life circumstances. Ultimately, success is not just about job titles or paychecks. It is about aligning your work with your values, strengths, and personal aspirations. By defining your own version of success—and having the courage to pursue it—you craft a career path that enriches your life and supports your overall well-being.

16.2 Clarifying Career Goals and Passions

Before making big decisions about your career, it helps to clarify what you truly want. Far too often, people chase goals set by family, society, or mere chance. To find a path that energizes and fulfills you:

1. **Self-Reflection**
   - **Likes and Dislikes**: Make a list of past jobs, school subjects, or personal projects. What did you enjoy or excel at? What bored or frustrated you?

- **Values**: Consider what matters deeply—helping others, creativity, independence, stability—and look for careers that align with those values.
2. **Skill Assessment**
    - **Hard Skills**: Technical abilities or specialized knowledge (like coding, accounting, writing).
    - **Soft Skills**: Communication, problem-solving, teamwork. Which come naturally to you, and which need improvement?
3. **Exploring Interests**
    - **Volunteer or Part-Time Work**: Trying small roles can reveal passions you never knew you had.
    - **Informational Interviews**: Talk to people in careers that interest you. Ask about their day-to-day tasks and what challenges or rewards they face.
4. **Dream Big, Then Filter**
    - **Brainstorm**: List all possible career paths you find intriguing—regardless of practicality.
    - **Refine**: Narrow it down based on feasibility, alignment with your strengths, and the potential lifestyle it offers.

Clarifying passions helps prevent wasted energy on jobs that do not suit you or keep you unhappy long-term. You may not find the perfect role overnight, but direction and experimentation bring you closer to your ideal fit.

16.3 Overcoming Gender Stereotypes in the Workplace

Women often face unspoken (and sometimes overt) stereotypes that can limit their career growth. Examples include assumptions that women are less capable in technical fields or are not serious about leadership because of family plans. To push back against these biases:

1. **Own Your Ambition**
    - **Confidence**: Speak openly about your career goals. Do not minimize your aspirations out of fear of appearing "pushy" or "too assertive."
    - **Supportive Network**: Surround yourself with people—mentors, colleagues—who believe in your potential.
2. **Confront Microaggressions Politely**

- **Examples**: If a coworker constantly interrupts you, calmly respond, "I'd like to finish my point first, please."
- **Documentation**: For repeated issues, keep written records, especially if biases are impacting your performance reviews or project assignments.

3. **Seek Allies**
   - **Team Up**: Look for coworkers who are open-minded, regardless of gender, who can amplify each other's voices during meetings.
   - **Employee Resource Groups**: If available, join or start groups for women in your industry, offering mutual support and advocacy.
4. **Professional Organizations**
   - **Networking**: Associations for women in engineering, law, business, etc., can provide resources, mentorship, and a sense of solidarity.
   - **Visibility**: By participating in conferences or speaking engagements, you showcase your expertise and break stereotypes.

While challenging stereotypes may feel daunting, steady, assertive action helps shift workplace culture over time. Each small act of standing up for yourself also bolsters your self-esteem, reminding you of your worth and abilities.

16.4 Building a Strong Professional Foundation

No matter your industry, you can lay the groundwork for long-term career success by focusing on these core areas:

1. **Continuous Learning**
   - **Formal Education**: Certifications, workshops, or advanced degrees can keep your knowledge updated.
   - **Informal Learning**: Online courses, webinars, or reading trade journals help you stay current on trends.
2. **Networking**
   - **Attend Industry Events**: Conferences, seminars, or local meetups can open doors to mentors, collaborators, or future employers.

      - **Social Media**: Platforms like LinkedIn enable you to connect globally, share insights, and learn from industry leaders.
3. **Personal Branding**
      - **Consistency**: Present a coherent image—your strengths, interests, and achievements—across resumes, social media, and personal interactions.
      - **Portfolio**: If relevant, maintain an online portfolio showcasing projects or samples of work.
4. **Work Ethic and Reliability**
      - **Reputation**: Being known as someone who meets deadlines, communicates clearly, and solves problems can lead to promotions or referrals.
      - **Professionalism**: Punctuality, respectful communication, and follow-through matter.
5. **Emotional Intelligence**
      - **Collaboration**: Successfully navigating different personalities can make you a valued team player or leader.
      - **Self-Awareness**: Recognize your emotional triggers at work, addressing them in healthy ways instead of letting them harm your performance or relationships.

These foundational elements stand out on a resume and in daily workplace interactions, setting you up for growth regardless of changing job markets or organizational shifts.

16.5 Handling Career Transitions

Career paths today are often fluid, with many women changing roles, industries, or starting ventures at different stages of life. If you find yourself contemplating a shift:

1. **Reevaluate Goals**
      - **Self-Check**: Ask, "Am I looking for a bigger salary, more creative freedom, or a better work-life balance?"
      - **Suitability**: Ensure the new direction lines up with your core values and current personal situation.
2. **Research Thoroughly**

- **Industry Insights**: Speak to people already in the field, read reports, or follow market trends to gauge future potential.
- **Skills Audit**: Identify gaps in your skills. Plan how to fill them through online courses, mentorships, or volunteer experiences.
3. **Financial Planning**
    - **Emergency Fund**: If you are leaving a stable job, have a safety net of savings to cover living expenses for several months.
    - **Gradual Transition**: Some women maintain their current role part-time while slowly building up a new endeavor, reducing financial stress.
4. **Emotional Preparation**
    - **Support System**: Inform friends, family, or a mentor about your plans so they can offer advice or moral support.
    - **Self-Belief**: Transitioning can be intimidating. Affirmations or journaling can keep negative self-talk in check.
5. **Test the Waters**
    - **Freelance or Side Projects**: Before fully committing, try short projects or part-time roles in the new field. This helps you confirm genuine interest.

A career transition can spark fresh motivation if done thoughtfully. Although challenging, it can ultimately lead to a role that matches your evolving interests and life situation.

16.6 Balancing Family and Career Demands

Many women face the challenge of juggling work with family roles—be it motherhood, caring for siblings, or supporting aging parents. Striking a balance is not always easy, but strategies can help:

1. **Set Boundaries at Work**
    - **Clarity**: Let your employer or team know when you are not available (e.g., certain evenings or weekends).
    - **Efficiency**: Use work hours effectively, minimizing distractions, so you can achieve more in less time.
2. **Seek Family Support**

- **Delegation**: *If you have a partner, split household tasks. Even children can do age-appropriate chores, teaching them responsibility.*
- **Communication**: *Discuss weekly schedules and needs with family so everyone is on the same page.*
3. **Employer Programs**
    - **Family-Friendly Policies**: *Some companies offer flexible schedules, remote work, or childcare assistance.*
    - **Negotiation**: *If policies are not clear, propose a pilot arrangement. Show how it can benefit productivity rather than hinder it.*
4. **Time Management**
    - **Prioritize**: *Not every task is equally important. Focus on what truly matters at home (e.g., family dinner, kids' events) while letting go of perfection in less critical areas.*
    - **Self-Care**: *Schedule short breaks for rest or personal enjoyment. A burnt-out caregiver or professional is less effective in both roles.*
5. **Let Go of Guilt**
    - **Reality**: *Trying to be a "perfect mom, perfect employee, perfect wife" can lead to constant stress.*
    - **Acceptance**: *Recognize that some days your career might need more attention; other days, family matters might take priority. It is a dynamic balance, not a static one.*

Achieving an ideal balance might be impossible every single day. Aim for a long-term equilibrium that honors your personal values, health, and relationships.

16.7 Facing Salary Negotiations and Promotions

Many women shy away from asking for a raise or promotion, fearing rejection or conflict. Yet standing up for fair compensation is important for career satisfaction. Tips to empower you:

1. **Do Your Research**
    - **Market Rates**: *Find out the standard salary range for your role and experience level in your region.*

- **Comparable Data**: Collect details like average salaries on job boards or surveys. This ensures your request is fact-based.
2. **Highlight Achievements**
    - **Proof**: Document specific ways you have added value—such as completing projects under budget, boosting sales, or improving team efficiency.
    - **Quantify**: Numbers speak loudly. Show percentages, revenue figures, or client satisfaction scores if applicable.
3. **Timing**
    - **Strategic Approach**: Schedule a meeting after a successful project or a positive performance review, when your accomplishments are fresh in your manager's mind.
    - **No Surprises**: Mention ahead of time that you want to discuss career growth or salary so your boss can prepare.
4. **State Your Number First**
    - **Anchor Technique**: If you open with a salary figure—based on research—it sets the range for discussion.
    - **Confidence**: Present your number clearly and calmly, without apologizing or seeming unsure.
5. **Collaborative Tone**
    - **Win-Win**: Emphasize how retaining you at a fair compensation benefits the organization (like stable leadership, project continuity).
    - **Alternative Perks**: If the company cannot increase salary immediately, consider negotiating extra vacation days, flexible hours, or professional development funds.

Securing the pay or role you deserve can significantly boost self-esteem and motivation. It also paves the way for future professional advancements.

16.8 Entrepreneurship and Small Business Ventures

If you have an entrepreneurial streak, starting your own business can be both thrilling and challenging. Women-owned businesses are growing worldwide, yet female entrepreneurs sometimes face unique obstacles—like difficulty accessing funding or managing family responsibilities. To succeed:

1. **Business Planning**

- **Market Analysis**: Identify a specific gap or need. Who are your target customers, and what problem do you solve for them?
- **Budget**: Outline start-up costs, ongoing expenses, and projected revenue. Seek advice from a trusted mentor or financial advisor if needed.

2. **Funding Options**
   - **Personal Savings**: Many entrepreneurs begin with their own funds, but it's wise to keep an emergency reserve.
   - **Loans or Grants**: Check local programs supporting women entrepreneurs, or explore small business loans from banks.
   - **Crowdfunding**: Platforms like Kickstarter can help you raise money if your idea resonates with the public.

3. **Lean Start-up Strategy**
   - **Test First**: Launch a minimum viable product or basic service to gauge market interest. This approach prevents large initial risks.
   - **Adapt Quickly**: Use feedback to refine your product or business model.

4. **Time Management**
   - **Wearing Many Hats**: Initially, you may handle marketing, finances, customer service, etc. Plan your schedule carefully to avoid burnout.
   - **Delegation**: As you grow, hire or contract professionals for tasks you are less skilled at—like accounting or social media management.

5. **Community Building**
   - **Networking**: Join local business associations or online forums for women entrepreneurs.
   - **Mentorship**: Finding an experienced business owner who can advise you saves time and prevents common mistakes.

While self-employment demands dedication, it can also offer immense creative freedom and the satisfaction of building something that reflects your vision and values.

16.9 Managing Workplace Challenges: Conflicts and Stress

Even in a fulfilling career, conflicts or stress can arise. Addressing problems early helps maintain a healthy work environment and protect your mental health:

1. **Conflict Resolution**
   - **Stay Objective**: Focus on the issue, not personal attacks. For example, "We have different views on how to handle this project. Let's list the pros and cons of each approach."
   - **Compromise**: Seek common ground. Sometimes a blend of both ideas is best.
2. **Handling Difficult Bosses or Coworkers**
   - **Professional Distance**: Keep interactions courteous and brief if someone is frequently negative. Document any serious issues like harassment.
   - **Seek Mediation**: If the relationship severely impacts your productivity or well-being, approach HR or a neutral party.
3. **Stress Management**
   - **Breaks**: Small breaks throughout the day—standing up, stretching, or deep breathing—reduce tension.
   - **Boundaries**: Try not to bring work conflicts home. Engage in after-work routines (like exercise or reading) to decompress.
   - **Speak Up**: If workload is excessive, talk to your manager about prioritizing tasks or distributing responsibilities.
4. **Emotional Health**
   - **Counseling**: In tough work environments, therapy can provide coping strategies and a safe space to process frustrations.
   - **Peer Support**: Confiding in a trusted colleague or friend can help you feel heard and validated.

Resolving or skillfully managing conflicts at work not only sustains your performance but also bolsters your confidence—knowing you can handle rough patches.

16.10 Mentorship and Sponsorship

Mentorship involves receiving guidance from someone with more experience, while sponsorship goes a step further—sponsors actively advocate for you, introducing you to opportunities or recommending you for roles. Both can be game-changers in a woman's career:

1. **Finding a Mentor**
    - **Identify Potential Mentors**: Look for individuals whose path or leadership style you admire.
    - **Reach Out Politely**: A concise email or personal approach can start the conversation. Mention what you hope to learn.
    - **Mutual Respect**: Be mindful of your mentor's time. Arrive prepared for meetings, and show appreciation for their insights.
2. **Gaining a Sponsor**
    - **High-Visibility Work**: Sponsors often notice people who excel in challenging or important projects.
    - **Relationship Building**: Sponsorship usually develops over time, as a senior figure sees your potential and decides to invest in your growth.
3. **Being a Good Mentee**
    - **Be Coachable**: Stay open to feedback, even if it challenges your comfort zone.
    - **Show Initiative**: Implement suggestions and give updates on your progress, demonstrating you value the mentor's advice.
4. **Pay It Forward**
    - **Future Mentoring**: As you advance, consider mentoring junior colleagues. This not only helps them but also refines your leadership skills.

Mentorship and sponsorship create supportive networks. Having someone who believes in your abilities can accelerate career success and keep you motivated.

16.11 Real-Life Example: Sara's Rise to Leadership

Sara began her career as a customer support agent in a tech firm. Initially, she struggled with self-doubt—thinking she might never climb the corporate ladder because she lacked a computer science degree. However, Sara made some strategic moves:

- **Continuous Learning**: She took free online courses on basic programming and tech terminology, enabling her to understand the product more deeply.
- **Excellent Work Ethic**: She gained a reputation for handling customer issues swiftly and going the extra mile to assist her teammates.
- **Seeking Mentors**: Sara reached out to a senior project manager, who taught her about product management and included her in important meetings.
- **Networking**: At company events, she introduced herself to key stakeholders. Over time, more people recognized her capabilities.
- **Stepping Up**: When a mid-level manager left abruptly, Sara volunteered to temporarily lead the support team. She proved her leadership skills, earning a promotion soon after.

Today, Sara holds a management position in that same company, guiding a team of 20 employees. She credits her rise to a mix of self-driven learning, seizing opportunities, and building strong relationships. Her story demonstrates how ambition, combined with a well-planned approach, can propel women to leadership roles—even when they start from a modest position.

16.12 The Role of Confidence in Career Growth

Confidence is not just a nice-to-have quality; it is crucial for:

1. **Assertive Communication**
    - **Meetings**: Confidently sharing your ideas or disagreeing respectfully can make you stand out as a thoughtful contributor.
    - **Email or Reports**: Writing with clarity and certainty shows you believe in your insights.
2. **Risk-Taking**
    - **Applying for Promotions**: Women sometimes wait until they match 100% of job criteria, whereas men apply earlier. Confidence helps you put yourself forward sooner.

        - **Starting Projects**: *Believing in your capacity to learn fosters innovation and creativity.*
3. **Handling Feedback**
        - **Growth Mindset**: *Confident individuals see criticism as a tool for improvement, not a personal attack.*
        - **Self-Advocacy**: *If feedback is unfair, confidence helps you speak up and clarify misunderstandings.*
4. **Leadership**
        - **Inspiring Others**: *A confident leader can motivate teams and instill trust in their vision.*
        - **Conflict Resolution**: *Being sure of your direction while remaining open to input balances authority with respect.*

If you lack workplace confidence, start small—volunteer for a minor project or share one idea in each team meeting. Overcoming initial nerves gradually builds the internal belief that your voice matters.

16.13 Lifelong Learning and Career Longevity

In a rapidly changing world, continuous learning can keep your career relevant and exciting:

1. **Stay Updated**
        - **Trends**: *Read about emerging tools, technologies, or methods in your field.*
        - **Micro-Courses**: *Many platforms offer short lessons you can fit into daily life—some are even free.*
2. **Diversify Skills**
        - **Complementary Talents**: *A writer might learn design basics, or a marketer might learn simple coding, making them more versatile.*
        - **Future-Proofing**: *Having multiple skill sets can protect you if one aspect of your job becomes automated or outdated.*
3. **Embrace Curiosity**
        - **Ask Questions**: *When you do not understand something, be willing to learn from teammates or attend workshops.*

- **Cross-Functional Collaboration**: Work with different departments to expand your understanding of how the whole company operates.
4. **Avoid Complacency**
    - **Reflect Regularly**: Ask, "Have I grown professionally this year? What skills do I want to gain next?"
    - **Certification Renewals**: If your field requires licenses or certifications, stay ahead of deadlines to maintain your qualifications.

Lifelong learning keeps you agile, ready for unexpected shifts, and invigorates your career with fresh perspectives.

16.14 Balancing Ambition with Personal Well-Being

High ambition can sometimes tip into overwork or burnout. To sustain performance, remember to care for your mental and physical health:

1. **Set Healthy Boundaries**
    - **Unplug**: Establish times when you do not check emails—like evenings or weekends.
    - **Vacation and Breaks**: Actual rest enhances long-term productivity and creativity.
2. **Watch for Burnout Signs**
    - **Symptoms**: Constant fatigue, irritability, or feeling detached from your tasks.
    - **Action**: Reassess workload, talk to a supervisor, or take a break to recharge before things worsen.
3. **Self-Care Routines**
    - **Physical Activity**: Regular exercise boosts energy and reduces stress hormones.
    - **Mindfulness**: Short daily meditations or stretches help clear mental clutter (linking back to Chapter 15's lessons).
4. **Celebrate Achievements**
    - **Recognition**: Acknowledge each promotion, project completion, or client success.
    - **Motivation**: Celebrating fosters gratitude and encourages you to keep striving without feeling perpetually unsatisfied.

Balancing drive with self-care ensures you do not sacrifice your health or happiness for career goals. A healthy approach can actually support greater career longevity and satisfaction.

16.15 Addressing Imposter Syndrome

Imposter syndrome is the feeling that you are not really as competent as others think, fearing you will be "found out" as a fraud. Many high-achieving women experience this, especially in male-dominated fields. To counteract it:

1. **Recognize It**
    - **Awareness**: *Notice patterns like discounting compliments ("They are just being nice") or attributing success to luck.*
    - **Separate Feelings from Facts**: *Remind yourself that your achievements are real and earned.*
2. **Challenge Negative Self-Talk**
    - **Evidence**: *List your accomplishments, skills, and positive feedback received.*
    - **Reality Check**: *Confide in trusted colleagues or mentors; they can reassure you that you are deserving of your role.*
3. **Accept Growth as Ongoing**
    - **Mindset**: *Realize that no one knows everything. Learning on the job does not mean you are inadequate—it means you are human and improving.*
    - **Mentorship**: *Even top leaders had mentors or made mistakes; you are not an exception for needing guidance.*
4. **Use Affirmations**
    - **Examples**: *"I am capable of handling new challenges," or "My work is valuable."*
    - **Consistency**: *Repeat them often, especially before high-pressure tasks like presentations or interviews.*

By gradually internalizing your accomplishments and allowing yourself to learn, you break free from the imposter syndrome's hold, stepping into roles with deserved confidence.

16.16 Crafting a Long-Term Career Vision

Beyond short-term goals like promotions or salary increases, having a broader vision helps guide your overall journey:

1. **Imagine Your Future Self**
   - **Prompt**: "Where do I see myself in 5, 10, or 20 years? What kind of work would I enjoy doing daily?"
   - **Lifestyle Considerations**: Factor in desired location, family plans, work-life balance, and financial goals.
2. **Set Milestones**
   - **Structured Roadmap**: Break down your vision into actionable steps—like acquiring certain certifications, expanding a professional network, or reaching a leadership position.
   - **Timelines**: Estimate how long each step might take, but stay flexible.
3. **Stay Adaptable**
   - **Expect Change**: You may discover new passions or face unexpected life events. Allow your vision to evolve.
   - **Frequent Check-Ins**: Every year or so, revisit your plan. Are you on track? Do you need to pivot?
4. **Emotional Motivation**
   - **Why**: Tying your vision to meaningful values—like wanting to mentor younger women or create innovative solutions—fuels commitment.
   - **Visuals**: Some people find inspiration in vision boards or journaling about future achievements.

A clear long-term vision acts like a compass. Even if the path winds, you have a sense of direction, making day-to-day decisions more purposeful.

16.17 Mentoring the Next Generation

As you progress, you may find opportunities to guide younger or less experienced women. Mentoring benefits both parties:

1. **Paying It Forward**
   - **Gratitude**: You likely received help along the way. Offering the same courtesy completes a cycle of support.

- **Legacy**: You shape a more inclusive and supportive work culture.
2. **Developing Leadership Skills**
    - **Teaching**: Clarifying concepts for someone else strengthens your own knowledge.
    - **Empathy**: Mentors learn to listen deeply and adapt their guidance to individual needs.
3. **Inspiring Confidence**
    - **Role Model**: Seeing a woman in a leadership or specialized role can encourage mentees to aim higher.
    - **Shared Experiences**: By sharing personal stories of failure and success, you show that challenges are normal and surmountable.

If formal mentorship programs are lacking, you can take smaller steps—like offering advice to an intern or inviting a junior colleague to shadow you for a day.

16.18 Realistic Measures of Success

Society often measures success with external markers—like a fancy title, a luxurious lifestyle, or social media "likes." But real fulfillment might differ:

1. **Personal Satisfaction**
    - **Question**: Do you wake up eager about your tasks more often than not?
    - **Indicator**: A sense of internal joy or purpose in your work, even if it is not glamorous from the outside.
2. **Positive Impact**
    - **Service**: Does your role improve others' lives, whether by solving problems or providing useful services?
    - **Legacy**: At the end of your career, will you feel proud of how you contributed to your community or field?
3. **Healthy Balance**
    - **Lifestyle**: Are you able to maintain friendships, family connections, and hobbies while pursuing your ambitions?
    - **Emotional Health**: Is your job adding to your stress or supporting your growth?

4. **Alignment with Values**
   - **Integrity**: You rarely have to compromise core morals or beliefs to succeed.
   - **Authenticity**: You can be yourself at work—open about your ideas and personality.

Assessing success on these deeper levels helps you avoid burnout or empty accomplishments. You build a career that is fulfilling on multiple dimensions, not just financially.

16.19 Maintaining Motivation Through Ups and Downs

Careers naturally ebb and flow. You might have periods of high motivation, followed by slumps. Sustaining drive requires:

1. **Short Sprints**
   - **Project-Based Goals**: Focus on completing a project with excellence, then rest or celebrate before starting another.
   - **Variety**: Rotate tasks or learn new skills to keep boredom at bay.
2. **Periodic Reflection**
   - **Check your "Why"**: Revisit why you chose this career and how it aligns with your life goals.
   - **Identify Burnout Signs**: If you feel constant fatigue or apathy, consider taking a break or discussing workload adjustments.
3. **Celebrating Small Wins**
   - **Reward System**: Treat yourself to something enjoyable—a day trip, a nice meal—after reaching milestones.
   - **Shared Success**: Publicly recognizing team achievements fosters collective motivation.
4. **Positive Peer Circles**
   - **Professional Groups**: Engaging with peers who share your aspirations keeps you inspired.
   - **Role Models**: Following stories of successful individuals can remind you that challenges are normal and can be overcome.

Understanding that career enthusiasm can fluctuate helps you plan for down times and re-energize your ambitions.

CHAPTER 17

Balancing Different Roles in Life

17.1 Introduction: The Many Hats Women Wear

Life can feel like a juggling act when you play multiple roles at once. You might be an employee, a manager, a mother, a daughter, a friend, a volunteer, a student—or any combination of these. Each role comes with its own set of responsibilities, expectations, and emotional demands. While some roles are chosen (like a career path), others arise naturally from life changes (such as becoming a parent or caregiver).

Balancing different roles can be fulfilling but also overwhelming. You may find yourself feeling guilty for giving more time to one area while another goes unnoticed. Or you may become exhausted by the mental and physical work of switching between roles so frequently. In this chapter, we will explore strategies to help you find a workable balance—or at least a healthier rhythm—so that you can fulfill multiple responsibilities without losing sight of your own well-being and personal growth.

17.2 Recognizing the Complexity of Multiple Roles

Each role you hold includes tasks, emotional demands, and sometimes conflicts with other roles. For instance, consider these examples:

- **Career and Parenthood**: You want to advance at work but also want to be present for your children's milestones.
- **Student and Family Caregiver**: You need time to study, yet family responsibilities eat into your study hours.
- **Entrepreneur and Volunteer**: Building a business is time-consuming, but volunteering is a passion you cannot ignore.

It is crucial to acknowledge this complexity. You are not "failing" if balancing is tough; it is inherently challenging. Give yourself permission to admit that *wearing multiple hats can be both rewarding and draining. Once you validate the difficulty, you can approach solutions with kindness and realism.*

17.3 Identifying Your Current Roles and Priorities

To achieve better balance, start by mapping out your existing roles. This might seem obvious, but many people carry extra responsibilities they do not fully account for. Here's a straightforward exercise:

1. **Make a Role Inventory**
    - **On Paper**: Write down all the roles you occupy—such as employee, entrepreneur, spouse, mother, friend, mentor, volunteer, daughter, homeowner, or student.
    - **Be Specific**: Some roles overlap. If you are an aunt who often babysits, that is a role worth noting.
2. **Rank or Categorize**
    - **High Priority**: Which roles are non-negotiable or central to your identity (e.g., taking care of a child)?
    - **Medium Priority**: Roles that matter but may be somewhat flexible (e.g., a hobby group or volunteer work).
    - **Low Priority**: Roles that you can reduce or delegate if needed (e.g., a social club you have joined out of habit rather than genuine interest).
3. **Reflect on Motivations**
    - **Ask "Why?"**: For each role, why do you maintain it? Do you love it, or do you feel obliged? Understanding motivations can reveal which roles are essential to keep and which might be adjusted.

This process clarifies how you currently spend your time and emotional energy. It also indicates where conflicts might arise—for instance, if two high-priority roles demand attention at the same time. Awareness is the first step in making strategic decisions about allocation of your resources.

17.4 The Myth of Perfect Balance

Our culture often promotes the idea of a "perfect work-life balance," as if there is a magical formula to distribute time evenly. However, the reality is more nuanced:

1. **Balance as a Dynamic Process**
   - **Changing Seasons**: Sometimes, your career may dominate—for instance, if you are launching a new business. Other times, family needs might take precedence, such as when caring for a newborn or an ailing relative.
   - **Fluid Shifts**: Balance might look different from one month to the next, and that is natural.
2. **Redefine Success**
   - **Individual Variation**: Each woman has unique priorities and constraints. A setup that works for your friend may not work for you.
   - **Quality Over Quantity**: Spending two focused hours with your child might be more meaningful than an entire day overshadowed by distractions or stress.
3. **Accept Imperfection**
   - **Letting Go of Guilt**: You cannot always give 100% to each role all the time. Sometimes you will miss an event or fall behind on a project. Forgiving yourself is crucial.
   - **Self-Compassion**: Rather than beating yourself up for not achieving perfect balance, recognize the effort you are making to juggle many responsibilities.

Viewing balance as an ongoing, evolving process helps you remain flexible, adjusting your focus based on current needs without feeling like a failure when things are not perfectly even.

17.5 Time Management Strategies for Multiple Roles

Although perfect balance is elusive, practical time management can reduce chaos and stress. Here are some helpful approaches:

1. **Block Scheduling**

- **Designated Slots**: Reserve specific blocks of time for certain roles. For example, 8:00 a.m. to 2:00 p.m. might be for work, 2:00 p.m. to 3:00 p.m. for family errands, and 3:00 p.m. to 5:00 p.m. for personal projects (if your schedule allows).
- **Clear Boundaries**: When in a given block, focus solely on that task or role. Avoid mixing work calls with family activities if possible.

2. **Prioritized To-Do Lists**
   - **Categorize Tasks**: Group tasks by role: "Work," "Family," "Personal," and rank them in order of urgency or importance.
   - **Daily or Weekly Approach**: Each morning or at the start of the week, decide on your top three priorities for each major role.

3. **Combine Roles When Appropriate**
   - **Overlap Wisely**: If you have older children, you might take a walk together while you discuss personal updates—fulfilling both "exercise" and "family bonding."
   - **Caution**: Overlapping roles can be efficient, but be mindful not to compromise quality. Some tasks demand exclusive focus.

4. **Use Technology**
   - **Shared Calendars**: Apps like Google Calendar let family members or coworkers see each other's schedules.
   - **Reminders and Alarms**: Automated alerts help you switch gears or recall important tasks.

5. **Delegate or Outsource**
   - **At Home**: If finances allow, hire help for cleaning or yard work. If you have a partner or older kids, divide tasks such as laundry or cooking.
   - **At Work**: If you lead a team, trust capable colleagues with tasks that do not require your personal input. Delegation fosters teamwork and eases your burden.

Good time management gives you the freedom to be present in each role, reducing mental clutter and that nagging sense of "I should be somewhere else."

17.6 Communication with Family and Colleagues

Balancing roles is easier when the people around you understand your situation and respect your boundaries:

1. **Explain Your Constraints**
   - **Family**: If you are nearing a big work deadline, let your spouse or kids know you need extra focus for a couple of days, then you will plan a special family activity.
   - **Work**: If you must leave early to care for a sick parent, inform your boss or team promptly. Most workplaces appreciate honesty and planning over last-minute surprises.
2. **Set Clear Expectations**
   - **Timelines**: At work, communicate realistic deadlines for your projects. At home, tell family members when you will be available for activities.
   - **Accessibility**: Decide if you will check work emails in the evening. If not, let colleagues know you will be offline after a certain hour.
3. **Negotiate Solutions**
   - **Compromise**: Talk with your partner about dividing responsibilities, or discuss flexible work arrangements with your employer.
   - **Flexibility**: Sometimes the solution might be a half-day remote work arrangement, or switching which parent picks up the kids from school on certain days.
4. **Use "I" Statements**
   - **Reducing Conflict**: If someone's demands clash with your schedule, calmly say, "I feel stressed when I cannot meet your expectations and mine. Can we find a middle ground?"
   - **Positive Framing**: Show you want to collaborate rather than accusing them of being inconsiderate.

Open, respectful communication helps you avoid hidden resentments or misunderstandings. It also makes others more willing to accommodate your multiple roles.

17.7 Coping with Role Conflicts

Despite best efforts, you will encounter role conflicts. A major work project might coincide with a family emergency, or a friend's celebration might fall on the same weekend you promised yourself rest. Here are ways to handle those conflicts:

1. **Evaluate Urgency**
   - **Critical vs. Optional**: If your child is sick, that likely takes priority over most work tasks, unless there is a truly non-moveable work crisis. On the other hand, if it is a routine event, maybe a trusted caregiver can fill in.
   - **Long-Term Effects**: Consider potential outcomes. Will skipping your friend's event damage the friendship irreparably, or can you make it up to them later?
2. **Seek Solutions Early**
   - **Proactive Approach**: If you see a conflict arising in the next month, start discussing solutions now rather than waiting until the last minute.
   - **Alternate Plans**: Maybe you can attend part of your friend's celebration or join virtually if you must travel for work.
3. **Make Peace with Imperfection**
   - **Reality**: Sometimes you cannot meet every obligation, and you might disappoint someone or feel disappointed.
   - **Apology and Understanding**: Express heartfelt regret if you must back out of something important. Offer to reconnect or compensate when you are more available.
4. **Reflect and Adjust**
   - **Lesson Learned**: Each conflict teaches you about your limits. Note if certain patterns keep recurring—like overcommitting on weekends or underestimating project timelines.
   - **Better Planning**: Use insights to plan future commitments more carefully.

Conflicts can be stressful, but handling them transparently and compassionately preserves relationships and self-respect.

17.8 Emotional Wellness: Avoiding Burnout

Burnout happens when constant demands from multiple roles overwhelm your mental, physical, and emotional capacity. Signs include chronic fatigue, irritability, cynicism, and lack of motivation. To protect against burnout:

1. **Monitor Your Stress Level**

- **Self-Awareness**: Check in with yourself daily or weekly. Do you feel consistently exhausted or restless?
- **Physical Clues**: Tension headaches, stomachaches, and recurring illnesses can indicate you are pushing too hard.

2. **Schedule Self-Care**
   - **Nonnegotiable**: Treat self-care—like exercise, relaxation techniques, or creative hobbies—as essential tasks, not optional luxuries.
   - **Micro-Breaks**: Even five-minute stretches or mindful breathing breaks can reset your mood.

3. **Mindful Boundaries**
   - **Saying No**: Politely decline extra responsibilities if you are near capacity, whether it is volunteering for another event or taking on additional chores at home.
   - **Digital Detox**: Limit time on social media or work email after hours. Constant connectivity can drain mental energy.

4. **Seek Help Early**
   - **Professional Support**: If signs of burnout intensify, consider therapy or counseling. A professional can provide tailored stress-management strategies.
   - **Delegation**: Talk to loved ones or coworkers about reassigning tasks during peak stress periods.

Catching burnout early can prevent more serious health or relationship issues down the road. Self-care is not selfish; it is a foundation for effectively handling all your roles.

17.9 Realistic Expectations and Letting Go of Perfection

Perfectionism can be especially crippling when balancing multiple roles. Trying to excel in each role at all times is unrealistic. Instead, aim for "good enough" where it truly matters:

1. **Identify Key Areas to Excel**
   - **Pinpoint**: Which roles or tasks genuinely require high precision—maybe a work project with tight standards or ensuring your kids' safety?
   - **Set a Standard**: Give your best in those high-impact areas.

2. **Accept "Good Enough" Elsewhere**
   - **Simplify**: Perhaps store-bought cookies for a bake sale are acceptable if you are short on time, instead of spending hours baking from scratch.
   - **Lower Pressure**: Reducing perfection in non-crucial tasks frees energy for what truly counts.
3. **Resist Comparison**
   - **Social Media Illusions**: Others might post pictures of elaborate birthday parties or immaculate homes, but you do not see the stress or resources behind the scenes.
   - **Personalized Approach**: Do what feels balanced for your context. Perhaps a small, heartfelt gathering works better than an extravagant event.
4. **Celebrate Small Wins**
   - **Gratitude**: Even if you did not achieve every item on your to-do list, note the tasks you completed or the role conflict you managed.
   - **Positive Reinforcement**: Acknowledging these successes encourages you to keep going without fixating on perceived "failures."

Letting go of the ideal of being the "perfect employee, perfect parent, perfect friend" can massively reduce stress. Embracing imperfections with grace can bring more joy to your daily life.

17.10 Involving Children in Household Responsibilities

If you are a parent, the family role can be one of the most time-intensive. Involving children in chores and decision-making not only alleviates your burden but also teaches them valuable skills:

1. **Age-Appropriate Tasks**
   - **Simple Jobs**: Younger kids can pick up toys or wipe tables, while older ones can help with laundry or cooking.
   - **Life Skills**: Children who learn responsibilities early often grow into more self-sufficient teenagers and adults.
2. **Make It Fun**

- **Team Effort**: Turn cleaning into a game or set a timer to beat the clock.
- **Music**: Play upbeat songs during chore time, creating a playful atmosphere.

3. **Explain Why**
    - **Contribution**: Show how each family member plays a role in keeping the household running. Emphasize teamwork rather than punishment or bribery.
    - **Confidence**: When children succeed in tasks, it boosts their self-esteem and sense of responsibility.
4. **Consistency**
    - **Schedules**: Assign regular chores (e.g., taking out trash every Tuesday).
    - **Praise**: Encourage them with positive feedback: "You did great organizing the bookshelf!"

By sharing household roles, you reduce the load on yourself and cultivate an environment where everyone learns cooperation and respect for each other's time.

17.11 Support Systems Outside the Home

Sometimes, external support can significantly help you manage various roles:

1. **Extended Family**
    - **Grandparents, Aunts, Uncles**: If they are willing and trustworthy, they can assist with childcare, errands, or emotional support.
    - **Reciprocal Arrangements**: You can offer to help them in return, creating a supportive family network.
2. **Friends and Community**
    - **Carpools and Babysitting Swaps**: Team up with neighbors or friends to share driving duties or take turns watching each other's kids.
    - **Local Organizations**: Community centers or places of worship may provide after-school programs, counseling, or social events that ease your responsibilities.
3. **Professional Services**

- **Daycare or Tutoring**: *If you have young children or are studying, professional childcare or tutoring can relieve some pressure.*
- **Meal Delivery or Housekeeping**: *Occasionally outsourcing these services might be worth the cost, especially during peak busy periods.*

4. **Support Groups**
   - **Parent Groups**: *Online or in-person networks where parents swap tips and moral support.*
   - **Caregiver Forums**: *If you care for an elderly parent, such communities offer resources, including respite care options.*

Expanding your support circle frees time and mental space, so you can better manage everything on your plate.

17.12 Tailoring Your Work Environment

If your workplace or business setting is rigid, balancing multiple roles can be more challenging. Look for ways to shape your environment:

1. **Flexible Schedules**
   - **Propose Alternatives**: *If feasible, ask about flex-time, compressed workweeks, or occasional remote work. Present a plan highlighting how it benefits productivity.*
   - **Core Hours**: *Some workplaces allow set "core hours" where everyone must be present, leaving the rest flexible.*
2. **Job-Sharing**
   - **Shared Role**: *In a job-share, two people split responsibilities of one full-time position. This arrangement is not common in all industries, but it can work well if both employees coordinate effectively.*
   - **Advantages**: *Job-sharing can reduce burnout and provide coverage during personal emergencies.*
3. **On-Site Amenities**
   - **Childcare**: *Some companies offer on-site daycare. If not available, suggest exploring such options.*

- **Wellness Programs**: *Gym access, meditation rooms, or mental health support can help employees handle stress from multiple roles.*
4. **Leadership Advocacy**
    - **Internal Influence**: *If you hold a senior position, you can advocate for policies that support work-life balance for everyone, like paid parental leave or mental health days.*
    - **Cultural Shift**: *Encouraging open discussions about life outside work reduces stigma around personal responsibilities.*

Adapting your work environment can improve not only your own balance but also workplace morale, leading to higher employee retention and satisfaction.

17.13 Transitioning Through Life Changes

Major life events—like marriage, divorce, a new baby, moving cities, or losing a loved one—disrupt existing balances. During transitions:

1. **Expect Temporary Imbalance**
    - **Adjustment Period**: *Understand that you may not maintain your usual routines for a while. This is normal.*
    - **Communication**: *Let friends, family, or coworkers know about the shift so they can understand any changes in your availability or mood.*
2. **Simplify**
    - **Prioritize**: *Reduce non-essential commitments until you stabilize. Focus on the crucial roles—such as a newborn's care—over less critical volunteer work.*
    - **Delegate More**: *Relatives or friends often want to help during big life changes, so let them pitch in.*
3. **Self-Care as a Priority**
    - **Mental Health**: *Consider counseling or support groups if you feel overwhelmed by grief or pressure.*
    - **Physical Health**: *Maintain basics like decent sleep, nutritious meals, and light exercise if possible.*
4. **Plan for the Next Phase**
    - **Gradual Return**: *Once the immediate upheaval eases, slowly reintroduce or shift focus to other roles.*

- **Reflection**: Life changes can alter your perspective on what matters. Reevaluate your role priorities and possibly pivot accordingly.

Periods of transition can feel chaotic, but they also bring opportunities for growth and redefinition of your life's balance.

17.14 Mindset Shifts for Sustainable Role Management

Beyond practical strategies, your mindset can drastically impact how you handle multiple roles:

1. **Growth Mindset**
   - **Learning Opportunity**: Each conflict or challenge is a chance to refine your skills—be it time management, negotiation, or emotional regulation.
   - **Adaptive Approach**: See setbacks as temporary, not permanent reflections of your ability.
2. **Resilience**
   - **Bouncing Back**: Cultivate the habit of bouncing back from mistakes or stressful weeks, rather than dwelling on regrets.
   - **Gratitude**: Pause to appreciate positives—a supportive friend, an understanding boss, or a child's progress—amid the juggling act.
3. **Self-Advocacy**
   - **Value Your Needs**: Recognize you have legitimate personal goals, not just obligations to others.
   - **Voice**: Speak up if roles become unmanageable. Request help, set boundaries, or negotiate changes.
4. **Compassion for Yourself and Others**
   - **Kindness**: Treat yourself with the same empathy you would offer a friend in a similar situation.
   - **Understanding**: Acknowledge that loved ones or coworkers also juggle multiple roles; mutual support fosters a more collaborative environment.

A mindset that embraces flexibility, resilience, and empathy can keep you afloat even when life's responsibilities intensify.

17.15 Real-Life Example: Beatrice's Balanced Approach

Beatrice works full-time in a sales role and is also a single mother of two school-aged kids. Initially, she felt guilty whenever she stayed late at the office, believing she was shortchanging her children. Then, guilt flipped when she left early for a child's recital, thinking her boss might see her as uncommitted to work. Constant stress made her snap at both coworkers and her kids.

After seeking advice from a friend, Beatrice made some changes:

- **Role Inventory**: She listed her roles—sales professional, mother, homeowner, church volunteer. She realized volunteering was optional and scaling back might relieve some stress.
- **Communicated with Her Boss**: She discussed her schedule, offering to arrive earlier on certain days so she could leave for school events without causing workflow problems. Her boss agreed once Beatrice demonstrated how she would still meet targets.
- **Family Meetings**: Every Sunday, Beatrice and her children planned the upcoming week. Her kids contributed to chores like packing lunches, and Beatrice promised each child one hour of uninterrupted "mom time" each weekday.
- **Self-Care Commitment**: She began waking 20 minutes earlier for a quick yoga session, which calmed her mind. She also set a weekend outing once a month purely for fun and relaxation with friends or family.
- **Evaluation**: She still had busy weeks, but less panic overall. She learned to forgive herself if everything did not go perfectly.

Beatrice's story shows how combining strategic communication, slight boundary shifts, and mindful scheduling can yield a healthier, more confident approach to juggling responsibilities.

17.16 Continuous Improvement in Balancing Roles

Balancing multiple roles is not a one-time fix; it requires ongoing adjustments:

1. **Periodic Check-Ins**
   - **Monthly or Quarterly**: Ask yourself, "Are my priorities still correct? Have I taken on any unnecessary roles?"
   - **Assess Stress Levels**: If stress is creeping up, revisit your schedule and consider whether another arrangement is needed.
2. **Flexible Mindset**
   - **Expect Shifts**: Kids grow, job demands evolve, your interests change. Roll with these shifts rather than resisting them.
   - **Reallocating Time**: As soon as you detect an imbalance—like too many late nights at work—rebalance by dropping or delegating tasks.
3. **Celebrate Achievements**
   - **Big and Small**: A promotion at work, your child excelling in school, or even smaller wins like a friend's birthday party you managed to attend.
   - **Positive Feedback Loop**: Recognizing successes encourages you to keep refining your approach without becoming disheartened by occasional setbacks.
4. **Plan for Future Growth**
   - **Skills Upgrades**: Maybe you want to learn better communication or delegation techniques to handle roles more effectively.
   - **Life Vision**: Keep an evolving picture of how you want your life to look in 5–10 years. Align your roles to support that vision.

Viewing role balance as a continuous improvement process allows you to evolve gracefully with changing circumstances and personal development.

17.17 Balancing Roles While Maintaining Relationships

Strong personal relationships and friendships can suffer when you are busy. To keep them healthy:

1. **Intentional Social Time**
   - **Scheduling**: Book a lunch date or short coffee meet-up with a friend weekly or monthly. If you do not plan it, it likely will not happen.

- **Technology**: *If distance is a barrier, arrange video calls with close friends or family members.*
2. **Quality Over Frequency**
    - **Deep Conversations**: *Even if you meet a friend less often, ensure you are present and engaged during those interactions.*
    - **Attentive Listening**: *Ask how they are doing, share updates about your life, and sincerely connect.*
3. **Combining Social and Functional**
    - **Errands Together**: *Grocery shopping or walking your dogs with a friend can serve dual purposes—catching up while completing tasks.*
    - **Family-Friends Mix**: *Host a casual gathering so your kids and friends can socialize too.*
4. **Set Relationship Boundaries**
    - **Saying "No" to Social Events**: *If you are already overwhelmed, politely decline or reschedule gatherings that are not crucial.*
    - **Honest Communication**: *Friends who truly care will respect your limited time if you explain your current situation.*

Nurturing relationships can provide emotional support, fun, and a sense of belonging—key ingredients for maintaining balance when life gets demanding.

17.18 Handling Cultural and Societal Pressures

Society and culture might push certain expectations—like women being primary caregivers, always available to family, or working unlimited hours to "prove" themselves. When cultural norms clash with your personal balance:

1. **Define Your Own Standards**
    - **Reflect**: *What do success and happiness look like to you personally, beyond societal ideals?*
    - **Self-Trust**: *Rely on inner convictions rather than external validation.*
2. **Selective Listening**
    - **Ignore Noise**: *If neighbors gossip about your parenting or your in-laws question why you work long hours, filter out unhelpful criticism.*

- **Value Constructive Feedback**: *If advice is well-meant and aligns with your core values, consider it. Otherwise, let it go.*
3. **Educate**
    - **Calm Explanations**: *Gently clarify your choices to family members with outdated views, like why you continue working after having kids.*
    - **Lead by Example**: *Over time, your results—happy children, a stable marriage, professional success—may challenge stereotypes more effectively than arguments.*
4. **Find Community**
    - **Like-Minded Circles**: *Seek peers who share your perspectives on balancing roles. They can offer solidarity and practical tips.*
    - **Support Groups**: *Online forums or local meetups exist for women defying cultural norms in areas like career or lifestyle.*

Standing up to societal or cultural pressures may be difficult but can bring great relief and empowerment once you set boundaries that honor your authentic needs.

17.19 Reinforcing Your Sense of Self

Amid the many roles, do not lose sight of who you are at your core. A strong self-concept protects you from being defined solely by any single role:

1. **Personal Identity Beyond Roles**
    - **Hobbies**: *Maintain at least one personal passion—like reading, painting, or hiking—that is purely for self-expression.*
    - **Values**: *Keep reminding yourself of key values such as honesty, creativity, empathy, or resilience.*
2. **Self-Reflection Practices**
    - **Journaling**: *Write about experiences in each role and how they affect your growth or emotions.*
    - **Mindfulness**: *Even brief daily sessions of focusing on your breath can ground you in your own being, apart from external demands.*
3. **Celebrating Individual Achievements**

- **Non-Role Achievements**: Recognize personal victories, like learning a new skill or overcoming a fear, unrelated to your professional or family roles.
- **Self-Validation**: Remind yourself that your worth is not solely based on what you do for others.

4. **Counseling or Coaching**
    - **Guidance**: If you struggle with identity issues—feeling lost among your roles—professional input can offer clarity.
    - **Objective Perspective**: A counselor can help you see patterns and suggest personalized coping strategies.

A strong inner sense of self helps you navigate role demands without losing authenticity or drowning in responsibilities.

CHAPTER 18

Mentoring and Guiding Others

18.1 Introduction: The Power of Lifting Others

Mentoring is more than just teaching someone a set of skills. It is about sharing wisdom, offering encouragement, and sometimes providing a friendly push when someone lacks confidence. Guiding others can be deeply rewarding, expanding your own sense of purpose and contributing to a supportive community. Whether you mentor a junior colleague at work, a family member stepping into adulthood, or a neighbor with less experience, your guidance can spark self-belief and success in someone else's life.

In this chapter, we will explore why mentoring and guiding others is beneficial for both the mentor and the mentee. You will learn how to establish a mentoring relationship built on respect and trust, adapt your teaching style to different personalities, handle common challenges, and celebrate growth milestones. Even if you do not see yourself as an expert, you have knowledge and perspectives that can help someone else. By stepping into a mentorship role, you reinforce your own confidence and play a vital role in building up the next generation of confident women.

18.2 Defining Mentorship and Its Importance

Mentorship involves a more experienced person (the mentor) supporting a less experienced one (the mentee) in navigating a particular domain—career, academics, personal growth, or any specialized area. Key characteristics of mentorship include:

1. **Guidance and Advice**
   - The mentor provides suggestions, strategies, and insights based on prior experience.
2. **Emotional Support**

- Beyond knowledge, mentors offer empathy, understanding, and encouragement during setbacks or self-doubt.
3. **Role Modeling**
    - Mentors demonstrate what is possible by sharing real stories of achievements, mistakes, and lessons learned.
4. **Long-Term Growth**
    - Rather than quick fixes, mentorship focuses on the mentee's overall development and self-sufficiency.
5. **Mutual Learning**
    - Mentors often discover new perspectives or keep up with trends through mentees, while mentees gain tools for success.

In many cultures and industries, mentorship has been pivotal in shaping leaders. By becoming a mentor, you contribute to that legacy, aiding progress while reinforcing your personal sense of purpose and leadership.

18.3 Benefits of Being a Mentor

Serving as a mentor can enrich your personal and professional life in numerous ways:

1. **Enhanced Leadership Skills**
    - **Communication**: You learn to explain concepts clearly, listen actively, and give constructive feedback.
    - **Empathy**: Helping someone through challenges teaches you to see the world from various perspectives.
2. **Self-Reflection**
    - **Reevaluating Knowledge**: As you teach others, you examine your own understanding, identifying gaps or clarifying complexities.
    - **Personal Growth**: Sharing your journey—failures and successes—can remind you of how far you have come, boosting confidence and gratitude.
3. **Expanded Network**
    - **Collaborative Bonds**: Mentees can become future colleagues, business partners, or references who champion your work.
    - **Reputation**: A reputation as a generous mentor can open doors and elevate your standing in your community or industry.

4. **Sense of Fulfillment**
   - **Purpose**: Watching someone succeed after you have helped guide them offers profound satisfaction.
   - **Paying It Forward**: You honor the mentors who once helped you, continuing the cycle of support.

By mentoring, you not only invest in someone else's future but also strengthen your own leadership and emotional intelligence.

18.4 Identifying Potential Mentees

You might wonder whom you could mentor. There are plenty of possibilities:

1. **Workplace Connections**
   - **New Hires**: If your company has interns or junior employees, you can volunteer to show them the ropes.
   - **Cross-Department**: You might guide someone in a different department who is curious about your field or skill set.
2. **Academic or Community Programs**
   - **School Partnerships**: Volunteer as a career speaker or a tutor. Younger students often benefit from seeing real-world examples of success.
   - **Nonprofits**: Many organizations run mentorship schemes, especially for marginalized groups or young women aiming to break into certain industries.
3. **Personal Networks**
   - **Family and Friends**: A cousin applying to college or a neighbor launching a small business might benefit from your advice.
   - **Online Platforms**: Social media or professional sites like LinkedIn can connect you with aspiring mentees seeking your expertise.
4. **Entrepreneurial Circles**
   - **Startup Incubators**: If you have experience in startups, you could help budding entrepreneurs refine their business models.
   - **Mastermind Groups**: A group of professionals can exchange knowledge, with more experienced members guiding newcomers.

Stay open to unexpected mentoring opportunities. Sometimes casual conversations or chance encounters reveal someone in need of exactly the insights you can provide.

18.5 Setting Up a Mentoring Relationship

While some mentorships happen informally, having structure can be beneficial:

1. **Initial Conversation**
   - **Clarify Expectations**: Ask the mentee about their goals—What do they hope to learn or achieve? Share what you can realistically offer.
   - **Match Personalities**: Ensure your styles align. A quiet mentee might need you to draw them out; an outspoken mentee might prefer more direct feedback.
2. **Agree on Format and Frequency**
   - **Meetings**: Decide whether to meet weekly, biweekly, or monthly, and if it will be in person or via video calls.
   - **Contact Methods**: Will you be available for quick questions via text or email between sessions?
3. **Set Boundaries**
   - **Time Commitments**: If you have limited availability, be honest. Overcommitting can strain both parties.
   - **Scope**: Define topics you feel comfortable guiding them on, and refer them to other resources for areas outside your expertise.
4. **Goals and Milestones**
   - **Short-Term**: Identify immediate skills or tasks the mentee wants to tackle.
   - **Long-Term**: Envision growth over a few months or a year. Encourage mentees to keep track of progress with specific, measurable milestones.

A structured beginning helps prevent misunderstandings. However, allow room for flexibility if goals evolve.

18.6 Effective Communication with a Mentee

Good communication builds trust and clarity:

1. **Active Listening**
   - **Techniques**: Maintain eye contact (if in person or video), ask follow-up questions, and summarize key points to confirm understanding.
   - **Avoid Interrupting**: Give the mentee space to express their ideas or frustrations before offering advice.
2. **Ask Open-Ended Questions**
   - **Encourage Reflection**: "What are your thoughts on this approach?" or "How do you feel about the feedback you received?"
   - **Empower Them**: Let the mentee discover answers rather than just giving a solution.
3. **Give Constructive Feedback**
   - **Specific and Kind**: Mention what was done well and where there is room for growth. Use examples.
   - **Solution-Focused**: Offer suggestions to improve, not just criticism. For example, "You might try practicing your presentation twice in front of a friend before the big day."
4. **Adapt to Their Style**
   - **Personality Sensitivity**: Some people prefer direct, to-the-point feedback; others need a gentler approach.
   - **Communication Medium**: If a mentee is shy about face-to-face discussions, allow them to ask questions via messages or email.

Honest, respectful communication not only helps mentees learn but also builds a strong mentor-mentee bond.

18.7 Guiding Mentees Through Challenges

Your mentee will inevitably face hurdles. A skilled mentor not only provides answers but also coaches them on problem-solving:

1. **Encourage Problem-Solving**

- **Ask "What if?"**: Instead of giving immediate solutions, say, "What do you think are possible ways to address this issue?"
            - **Support Brainstorming**: Let them list multiple options, and then discuss pros and cons together.
    2. **Validate Feelings**
        - **Empathy**: Acknowledge their frustration, fear, or disappointment. "I understand this must be stressful for you."
        - **Optimism**: Offer reassurance that setbacks are normal and do not define their capabilities.
    3. **Share Personal Experiences**
        - **Relatable Stories**: Briefly describe a similar challenge you faced. Emphasize the lessons learned, not just your success.
        - **Authenticity**: If you made mistakes, admit them. This humanizes you and shows them resilience.
    4. **Suggest Resources**
        - **Professional Help**: If the problem goes beyond your scope—like severe anxiety—encourage them to see a counselor or other experts.
        - **Books or Workshops**: Recommend relevant materials or training sessions that can deepen their knowledge.

Guiding a mentee through obstacles builds their confidence and resilience, teaching them that challenges are stepping stones rather than dead ends.

18.8 Balancing Support and Independence

An effective mentor-mentee relationship strikes a balance: you provide guidance without micromanaging or stifling the mentee's autonomy:

1. **Empower Decision-Making**
    - **Promote Ownership**: Let the mentee decide which advice to follow. Respect their choices, even if they differ from yours.
    - **Self-Reliance**: Encourage them to gather information and weigh options, so they become problem-solvers in the long run.
2. **Resist Doing Tasks for Them**
    - **Hands-Off Approach**: Offer pointers, but do not take over. If they are learning a skill—like writing a business plan—guide them, but let them draft it.

- **Confidence Building**: Each time they solve a problem independently, their confidence grows.
3. **Check-Ins**
    - **Progress Updates**: Periodically ask how they are doing. Are they stuck or do they need a new perspective?
    - **Measured Intervals**: Step in more actively only if you see them floundering with no progress or repeating the same mistakes without learning.

When mentees develop independence, they grow stronger and more resourceful, which is the true goal of mentorship.

18.9 Group Mentoring and Peer Circles

While traditional mentorship is often one-on-one, group mentoring models also provide rich experiences:

1. **Mentoring Circles**
    - **Structure**: A small group of mentees meets with one or more mentors. Everyone shares experiences, insights, and support.
    - **Diverse Perspectives**: Each mentee brings different backgrounds and challenges, offering varied learning points.
2. **Peer Mentorship**
    - **Equal Footing**: In some cases, peers at a similar career or life stage help each other, exchanging skills and holding each other accountable.
    - **Rotational Learning**: Each participant might lead a session on their strong area, fostering collective knowledge-building.
3. **Online Forums**
    - **Accessibility**: Virtual groups allow mentorship beyond geographic boundaries.
    - **International Insights**: Members can learn about different cultural or industry practices, broadening their horizons.

These collaborative formats encourage community spirit and reduce the mentor's burden by distributing support among several participants.

18.10 Special Considerations for Women Mentoring Women

While anyone can mentor anyone else, there is a unique power when women mentor other women, especially in male-dominated fields:

1. **Shared Experiences**
   - **Understanding Gender Bias**: A female mentor can empathize with issues like work-family balance or encountering subtle sexism in the workplace.
   - **Practical Tips**: Learning how other women overcame these barriers can guide a mentee's approach to dealing with similar challenges.
2. **Role Modeling**
   - **Representation**: Seeing a woman excel in leadership or specialized roles can inspire younger women to believe in their potential.
   - **Empowerment**: A female mentor can actively challenge societal norms that discourage women from ambition.
3. **Safe Space**
   - **Open Dialogue**: Women might feel more comfortable discussing sensitive topics—like workplace harassment or maternity concerns—with another woman who has navigated them.
   - **Encouraging Confidence**: Mentors can specifically target issues like imposter syndrome or negotiation hesitancies that many women face.

Women supporting women creates a ripple effect, strengthening entire communities. Each mentee can become a future mentor, perpetuating the cycle of empowerment.

18.11 Navigating Cultural and Personality Differences

Mentoring relationships can cross cultures, generations, or personality types. Adapting to differences is vital:

1. **Cultural Sensitivity**

- **Learn About Backgrounds**: Ask mentees about their cultural norms or values to avoid misunderstandings.
- **Inclusive Language**: Be aware of possible language barriers or differing communication styles.

2. **Generational Gaps**
   - **Technology Use**: Younger mentees may rely heavily on digital tools, so be open to learning from them.
   - **Communication Preferences**: Some older mentees might prefer phone calls over texts, or vice versa.
3. **Personality Styles**
   - **Introverted vs. Extroverted**: An introverted mentee may need more gentle prompting, while an extroverted one might thrive on lively debates.
   - **Analytical vs. Creative**: Adjust examples or problem-solving approaches to match how they process information.

Embracing diversity within mentor-mentee relationships fosters richer learning experiences for both parties.

18.12 Handling Mentorship Challenges

Mentorship is not always smooth:

1. **Lack of Commitment**
   - **Mentee Issues**: If a mentee repeatedly cancels meetings or does not follow through, gently but firmly address it. Ask if something is blocking their engagement.
   - **Mentor Boundaries**: If it continues, you may limit your involvement or step away, as forcing mentorship rarely works.
2. **Personality Clashes**
   - **Identify Conflicts**: If you sense tension—maybe mismatched communication styles—bring it up kindly: "I notice we're struggling to understand each other. How can we adjust?"
   - **Mediation**: If in a corporate program, an HR or program coordinator might help resolve deeper conflicts.
3. **Overdependence**

- **Encourage Autonomy**: If the mentee leans on you for every little decision, redirect them to make smaller calls independently.
- **Reassert Boundaries**: Remind them you are not always available and that part of growth is self-reliance.

4. **Life Changes**
   - **Transitions**: If the mentee moves to a different city or you change jobs, you might need to adapt meeting formats or end formal mentorship on good terms.
   - **Closure or Continuation**: Decide together whether to continue a looser arrangement via monthly calls or end the mentorship if it no longer serves the mentee's goals.

Openly discussing issues can salvage many mentorships, and parting ways respectfully is always better than letting a relationship fizzle or turn sour.

18.13 Encouraging Mentees to Mentor Others

Part of building a supportive community is inspiring mentees to pay it forward:

1. **Highlight Their Strengths**
   - **Confidence Boost**: Remind them that they have valuable insights to share, even if they are still learning.
   - **Small Steps**: Suggest they answer beginners' questions in online forums or assist a new coworker.
2. **Model Humility and Collaboration**
   - **Openness**: Show that you, too, learn from others and are not the sole authority.
   - **Shared Platform**: In group settings, invite your mentee to share their experiences or solutions.
3. **Offer Support**
   - **Transition**: If your mentee is ready, encourage them to start mentoring someone, and assure them you will be there if they need guidance on how to mentor.
   - **Resources**: Provide reading materials or tips on effective mentorship so they feel equipped.

Planting the idea of mentorship in your mentee's mind helps expand the culture of mutual help—ensuring that knowledge and encouragement flow to the next wave of learners.

18.14 The Relationship Between Mentorship and Leadership

Mentorship is often viewed as a leadership skill:

1. **Developing Leadership Qualities**
   - **Vision and Guidance**: Mentors guide mentees toward a bigger picture, similar to how leaders direct teams.
   - **Inspiring Trust**: Good mentors earn trust through consistency and empathy, a hallmark of effective leaders.
2. **Team Building**
   - **Stronger Organizations**: In workplaces where senior staff mentor junior members, the overall team grows more competent and cohesive.
   - **Succession Planning**: Mentorship prepares the next generation of leaders, ensuring continuity when older leaders retire or move on.
3. **Reputation and Influence**
   - **Credibility**: Recognized mentors are seen as supportive and skilled, making them respected within organizations.
   - **Positive Culture**: Mentoring fosters an environment of shared learning rather than cutthroat competition.

Leaders who invest in mentorship demonstrate a commitment to collective growth, which can inspire loyalty and drive innovation.

18.15 Real-Life Example: Tasha's Mentorship Journey

Tasha began working in a large manufacturing company as a data analyst. Over time, she became proficient in interpreting complex data, streamlining production reports, and delivering clear presentations. Feeling grateful for her own mentors, she decided to mentor a junior analyst, Sophia.

- **Early Stage**: They agreed to meet biweekly. Tasha asked Sophia about her career goals—she aimed to eventually lead data projects but lacked confidence in her technical communication.
- **Guidance**: Tasha taught Sophia how to simplify data points for presentations, offered sample slides from past projects, and introduced her to key internal stakeholders.
- **Challenges**: Sophia often hesitated to give her opinions in team meetings, fearing she was "too new." Tasha encouraged her to share at least one idea per meeting and praised her efforts each time.
- **Progress**: Within six months, Sophia delivered a short but impactful presentation on a new data model. Management noticed her potential, and she was invited onto a special task force.
- **Paying It Forward**: Inspired by Tasha's support, Sophia began informally guiding two new interns, helping them interpret basic data and navigate the company's culture.

Through this journey, Tasha refined her own communication skills—she realized that teaching concepts clarified them in her own mind. Sophia, in turn, gained confidence and soon passed that confidence along to interns. Their story reflects how mentorship can create a chain reaction of growth.

18.16 Celebrating Mentees' Achievements

Nothing boosts a mentee's morale like recognition from a respected mentor:

1. **Public Acknowledgment**
    - **Group Settings**: If appropriate, congratulate them during team meetings or on social media for a job well done.
    - **Crediting Efforts**: Emphasize their hard work and personal initiative rather than making it sound like your mentorship did everything.
2. **Private Encouragement**
    - **Personal Note**: Send them a heartfelt email or card praising a milestone—like acing a test or completing a challenging project.
    - **One-on-One Chat**: Let them know you are proud, reinforcing that you noticed their dedication.
3. **Reflecting on Growth**

- **Progress Recap**: *Periodically remind them where they started and how far they have come.*
- **Next Steps**: *Use a success as a springboard for discussing future ambitions.*

Celebrating mentees fosters motivation and resilience, showing them that each achievement is a step toward larger goals.

18.17 Mentoring Across Different Life Stages

Mentorship is not limited to early-career individuals; it can be valuable at any stage:

1. **Teenagers and Young Adults**
    - **Career Exposure**: *Help them explore potential paths and prepare for the transition to higher education or initial employment.*
    - **Life Skills**: *Topics like financial literacy, time management, and relationship building can be crucial.*
2. **Mid-Career Professionals**
    - **Upgrading Skills**: *Mentors can guide them on leadership development or specialized knowledge to shift into new roles.*
    - **Work-Life Balance**: *Advice on managing family or personal commitments with career progression is invaluable.*
3. **People Returning After a Break**
    - **Career Gaps**: *Women returning from maternity leave or a hiatus might need help updating skills or adjusting to workplace changes.*
    - **Confidence Rebuilding**: *Assurance that their past experience remains valid and beneficial helps them reintegrate smoothly.*
4. **Late-Career Transitions**
    - **Legacy and Mentorship**: *Seasoned professionals may want guidance on transitioning to part-time consulting, volunteering, or new industries.*
    - **Purpose**: *Mentoring helps them find continued meaning even beyond traditional retirement.*

No matter the age or stage, supportive guidance fuels personal and professional growth.

18.18 Self-Care for Mentors

While mentoring is fulfilling, it requires emotional energy and time:

1. **Set Boundaries**
   - **Availability**: Decide how frequently you can meet or respond to messages. Overextending can breed burnout.
   - **Scope**: If mentees ask for help outside your expertise or comfort level, point them to relevant resources instead of trying to handle it all.
2. **Allocate "You" Time**
   - **Balance**: Do not let mentoring overshadow your own goals or family responsibilities.
   - **Scheduled Breaks**: If you are mentoring multiple people, plan downtime to recharge mentally.
3. **Seek Support**
   - **Peer Mentors**: Connect with other mentors to swap ideas, discuss challenges, and share best practices.
   - **Celebrate Success**: Give yourself credit for the difference you are making, acknowledging your dedication and empathy.

Maintaining your well-being ensures you can continue mentoring effectively without sacrificing your personal life or health.

18.19 Transitioning or Concluding a Mentoring Relationship

Sometimes, mentorships naturally wind down:

1. **Milestone Completion**
   - **Goal Achievement**: If the mentee has reached a major objective—like landing their dream job—the formal mentorship might no longer be needed.

- **Celebration**: Mark this transition with a final meeting, congratulating them on their accomplishment.
2. **Reduced Contact**
    - **Periodic Check-In**: You might move from regular sessions to an occasional email update or coffee catch-up.
    - **Open Door**: Let them know they can reach out for future guidance if needed.
3. **Fading Out**
    - **Change in Circumstances**: If either party changes location or priorities, mentorship might taper off.
    - **Respectful Goodbye**: Communicate clearly rather than simply vanishing. Express appreciation for the journey.

Ending a mentorship relationship on a positive note maintains goodwill. Mentees often remain part of your network, and you might reconnect down the line.

CHAPTER 19

Crafting a Personal Development Plan

19.1 Introduction: The Value of a Clear Roadmap

For many women, confidence arises not just from random successes but from having a sense of direction and ownership over personal growth. A personal development plan (PDP) is like a roadmap guiding you toward the best version of yourself. While you cannot predict every twist and turn of life, having a plan helps you focus on goals that align with your values, strengths, and dreams. It turns broad desires—like "I want to feel more accomplished" or "I want to build my skills"—into specific, actionable steps you can track.

In this chapter, you will learn how to design a personal development plan that is realistic, motivating, and easy to follow. You will discover methods for setting priorities, measuring progress, and staying adaptable. Even if you have never made a formal plan before, this step-by-step approach will show you that developing confidence and personal fulfillment can be structured in a clear, intentional way. Rather than drifting through life hoping for change, you can actively shape your journey and celebrate each milestone along the path.

19.2 Understanding What a Personal Development Plan Is

A personal development plan is a written (or digital) document outlining your goals, the actions you will take to reach them, and the timeframe for each step. It also includes ways to track and evaluate your progress. While it is not a rigid contract, it acts as a guiding framework. Common elements include:

1. **Goals and Aspirations**
    - **Definition**: Simple statements of what you want to achieve—like "Improve my public speaking skills," "Launch a small online business," or "Build stronger relationships."

- **Variety**: You might set professional goals (career advancement), personal goals (health or creative hobbies), or relationship goals (family bonding).
2. **Action Steps**
    - **Concrete Tasks**: Break each goal into smaller tasks. For instance, if your goal is to be a better public speaker, tasks could include "Join a local Toastmasters club" or "Practice a presentation in front of friends."
    - **Resources**: Identify the books, courses, or mentors who can help you learn faster.
3. **Timeline and Milestones**
    - **Deadline**: Without a rough timeline, you risk procrastination or losing motivation. Specify a target date for each milestone.
    - **Checkpoints**: Plan for periodic reviews—like every month or quarter—to evaluate if you are on schedule or need adjustments.
4. **Measurement and Evaluation**
    - **Key Indicators**: Decide how you will measure success. For instance, if you aim to save money, define the exact amount you want in your savings account by a certain date.
    - **Reflection**: Keep notes or a journal. After each checkpoint, record what worked, what did not, and how you feel.
5. **Adaptability**
    - **Flexibility**: Life changes, so allow room to modify your plan. A personal development plan evolves with you, not the other way around.

By clarifying your hopes into clear, measurable goals, you give yourself a powerful tool to stay focused and build true self-confidence over time.

19.3 Laying the Foundation: Reflecting on Your Values and Strengths

Before you jump into listing goals, take time to understand who you are at a deeper level. Reflecting on your values, strengths, and passions ensures your plan aligns with what truly matters to you:

1. **Identify Core Values**

- **Examples**: Honesty, creativity, family, independence, compassion, growth, service, or adventure.
- **Process**: Think about moments you felt most fulfilled or upset—these experiences often reveal your core values. If you felt angry over injustice, "fairness" might be a key value. If you glowed with joy after helping a friend, "generosity" could be central.

2. **Explore Strengths and Natural Talents**
   - **Current Skills**: Are you good at organizing, writing, listening, or problem-solving?
   - **Positive Feedback**: Ask friends or coworkers what they see as your best qualities or talents. Sometimes they spot strengths you overlook.
3. **Recognize Personal Passions**
   - **Hobbies and Interests**: Which activities excite you, make time fly, or spark your creativity?
   - **Causes and Projects**: Do you feel drawn to volunteer work, environmental issues, or entrepreneurial ideas?
4. **Assess Life Satisfaction**
   - **Wheel of Life**: Some people use a "Wheel of Life," dividing areas like career, health, relationships, finances, personal growth, fun, etc. Rate each area from 1 to 10. This exercise reveals which areas might need more attention in your personal development plan.

Understanding these foundational elements guides you to set goals that resonate. For instance, if "creativity" is a top value but your daily life allows no creative outlet, your plan might include learning an instrument, painting once a week, or writing short stories. Feeling aligned with your values fosters motivation and ensures your goals truly enhance your life.

19.4 Deciding Which Goals to Include in Your Plan

You might have a dozen ambitions—improving communication, learning a new language, getting fit, starting a nonprofit, or boosting financial literacy. Attempting them all at once can dilute your focus. A well-structured personal development plan prioritizes a few key goals at a time.

1. **Narrow Your Goals**
   - **Core Objectives**: Pick a manageable number—maybe three to five—for your first cycle of planning. Spreading yourself too thin can lead to frustration.
   - **Impact and Feasibility**: Evaluate which goals will bring the greatest impact on your overall well-being. Also consider how practical they are given your resources and current life demands.
2. **Balance Different Life Areas**
   - **Holistic Approach**: Ideally, your goals should touch different facets of life, such as professional, personal, health, and relationships. That way, you grow in multiple dimensions.
   - **Avoid Overloading**: If your career is very demanding now, maybe choose a smaller personal hobby goal rather than a massive new project.
3. **Timeframe**
   - **Short-Term vs. Long-Term**: Include both types. A short-term goal might be "Master a basic yoga routine within three months," while a long-term goal might be "Achieve a management position within three years."
   - **Staggering Start Dates**: If your goals are large, consider starting them at different times, so you do not become overwhelmed.
4. **SMART Method**
   - **Specific**: Instead of "get in shape," say "attend a 30-minute dance class twice a week."
   - **Measurable**: Track how often you achieve that, or see how your stamina improves.
   - **Achievable**: Ensure it is realistic given your schedule or fitness level.
   - **Relevant**: Does it match your values—like health or self-expression?
   - **Time-Bound**: Set an end date or milestone markers.

Focusing on a select set of meaningful goals helps you channel your energy effectively and build confidence as you see real progress.

19.5 Breaking Down Goals into Action Steps

Large or long-term goals can feel daunting, but breaking them into bite-sized tasks makes them doable:

1. **From Goal to Tasks**
   - **Brainstorm**: If your goal is "Start a side business selling handmade crafts," list everything needed—like setting up social media pages, designing product samples, researching shipping, etc.
   - **Sequence**: Organize the tasks in logical order. For example, you might first decide on your brand name and logo before creating an online shop.
2. **Realistic Timelines**
   - **Estimates**: Decide how much time each step requires. If "Build a website" is a 10-hour task, schedule it accordingly.
   - **Buffer**: Add extra time for learning curves or unforeseen issues. Life rarely goes exactly as planned.
3. **Prioritize Tasks**
   - **Order of Impact**: If certain tasks have a bigger effect, do those first.
   - **Dependencies**: Some tasks cannot start until others are completed—like you cannot order business cards before finalizing your brand name.
4. **Daily and Weekly Micro-Actions**
   - **Small Steps**: Break tasks further into daily or weekly goals. For instance, "Research two website platforms by Friday," or "Write a first draft of my business plan by next Tuesday."
   - **Visibility**: Put these micro-goals on a calendar or to-do list so you see them regularly.

By chunking big ambitions into step-by-step tasks, you reduce overwhelm. Each completed task also provides a mini victory that fuels motivation and confidence.

19.6 Creating a Timeline and Setting Milestones

Clear timelines keep you focused and prevent constant procrastination:

1. **Overall Timeline**
   - **Time Span**: Decide if your personal development plan covers 3 months, 6 months, or a year. Some people prefer quarterly cycles, while others do a yearly plan with monthly checkpoints.
   - **Reasonable Pace**: Set deadlines that push you to act but are still achievable given work, family, and personal obligations.
2. **Milestones and Checkpoints**
   - **Mini-Deadlines**: For each goal, identify specific points marking progress. For example, if your goal is to write a novel, a milestone might be completing a chapter outline, then finishing the first three chapters, etc.
   - **Reward System**: Plan small rewards for hitting milestones. This could be a relaxing bath, a nice meal, or even sharing your success with a supportive friend.
3. **Flexibility and Reevaluation**
   - **Life Happens**: If a family emergency arises, you might adjust your deadlines. That does not mean you have failed; it means you are practical.
   - **Regular Reviews**: Once a month (or more often), reflect on your progress. If you are consistently missing deadlines, investigate why. Are they unrealistic, or did you overcommit?

A timeline combined with milestones transforms vague plans into concrete targets, keeping you steadily on course and giving you tangible points to celebrate along the way.

19.7 Tracking Progress and Staying Motivated

Even the best plan can fizzle if you do not monitor progress or renew your motivation:

1. **Progress Journals and Checklists**
   - **Daily or Weekly Notes**: Keep track of completed actions and any insights. This helps you spot patterns—like repeated delays—or celebrate consistent effort.
   - **Digital Tools**: Use apps that log your tasks or send reminders. Trello, Asana, or even a basic spreadsheet can work.
2. **Regular Reflections**

- **Structured Questions**: Ask yourself weekly, "What went well?" "What was challenging?" "Do I need to adjust something?"
 - **Emotional Check**: Are you still enjoying this journey, or is the pressure too high? Sometimes a small tweak—like working on your goal earlier in the day—improves your mood.
3. **Stay Inspired**
 - **Visual Reminders**: Some people create vision boards or place sticky notes with encouraging words around their workspace.
 - **Success Stories**: Read or listen to others who achieved similar goals. Their stories can rekindle your excitement and remind you that it is possible.
4. **Accountability Partners**
 - **Buddy System**: If you know someone with a similar ambition (like improving health or studying for an exam), update each other regularly.
 - **Mentor or Coach**: Paying for a life coach or seeking a mentor can add structure and professional advice to keep you on track.

When you observe small wins—like finishing a specific task or receiving positive feedback—take a moment to appreciate your dedication. Regular acknowledgment fosters ongoing motivation.

19.8 Overcoming Obstacles and Setbacks

No personal development plan goes perfectly. Obstacles—like time constraints, unexpected events, or self-doubt—will appear. The key is addressing them head-on:

1. **Identify Common Roadblocks**
 - **Time Crunch**: Maybe you underestimated how busy your weekends would be.
 - **Emotional Fatigue**: Perhaps you feel too drained after work to study or exercise.
 - **Resource Shortage**: You cannot afford a course you planned, or you lack transportation for an activity.
2. **Brainstorm Solutions**
 - **Time Management Tweaks**: Simplify your approach, delegate tasks, or switch to a shorter daily routine.

- **Emotional Self-Care**: Add small pockets of relaxation—like a quick nap, mindful breathing, or a chat with a supportive friend.
- **Alternative Resources**: If you cannot pay for a course, search for free online materials or community workshops.

3. **Seek Support Early**
   - **Mentors and Coaches**: They can offer fresh strategies or connect you with relevant contacts.
   - **Friends and Family**: Be open about your challenges. Sometimes a friend's advice or assistance—like babysitting while you study—can save a plan.

4. **Adjust the Plan If Needed**
   - **Scaling Back**: If your initial goal was too big for the current season of life, reduce or modify it. Better to achieve a scaled version than to abandon it entirely.
   - **Extending Timelines**: If you just need a little more time, push a deadline by a couple of weeks.

Overcoming setbacks actually strengthens your confidence. Each time you navigate a hurdle, you prove your resilience and adaptability, which are central to genuine self-belief.

19.9 The Role of Reflection and Self-Awareness

A personal development plan is not just about reaching a destination; it is about understanding yourself more deeply through the journey:

1. **Regular Self-Check-Ins**
   - **Emotional State**: Are you genuinely happy pursuing these goals, or are you going through the motions? Check if the plan still resonates with your core values.
   - **Learning from Mistakes**: Each obstacle or misstep can reveal something about your habits, triggers, and preferences.

2. **Evolving Identity**
   - **Shifting Values**: As you grow, your priorities may change. For instance, a career-driven goal may be replaced by a new interest in creative arts.

- **Confidence Building**: Observing your capacity to adapt and learn fosters a stronger self-image.
3. **Journaling for Clarity**
    - **Written Reflections**: Spend a few minutes writing about your experiences, breakthroughs, and questions. This process often clarifies hidden feelings or potential solutions.
    - **Guiding Questions**: "What did I learn this week?" "What am I grateful for?" "How has this experience changed my perspective?"
4. **Accountability to Yourself**
    - **Honesty**: You are your own best motivator if you remain truthful about your progress or lack thereof.
    - **Self-Celebration**: Even small improvements, like waking up 30 minutes earlier to read a motivational book, are steps forward.

Reflection ensures your personal development plan remains meaningful, dynamic, and aligned with who you are becoming.

19.10 Celebrating Milestones and Adjusting the Plan

Completion of a milestone is not the end of the journey—it is a chance to celebrate, regroup, and move forward:

1. **Marking Success**
    - **Small Rewards**: Treat yourself after a milestone. Examples: a relaxing spa day, a new journal, or a trip to your favorite coffee shop.
    - **Public Acknowledgment**: Share your accomplishment with a supportive friend, family member, or on social media if you feel comfortable.
2. **Plan Review**
    - **Assess the Next Steps**: After reaching one milestone, see if the next steps remain the same or need updates based on new insights.
    - **Reevaluate Deadlines**: If you finished early or late, adjust future timelines accordingly.
3. **Refining Goals**

- **Changing Priorities**: *If something else in your life has become more pressing, reorder your goals.*
- **New Opportunities**: *Maybe an unexpected chance—like an invitation to join a community project—sparks a new goal.*

4. **Gratitude and Confidence**
   - **Reflect**: *Acknowledge how far you have come. This sense of achievement builds confidence for tackling further challenges.*
   - **Stay Humble**: *Recognize that there is always more to learn, but you have the ability to keep progressing.*

By treating milestones as checkpoints rather than finish lines, you maintain momentum and an ongoing sense of fulfillment.

19.11 Examples of Personal Development Goals

If you are unsure where to start, consider these broad goal areas and adapt them to your context:

1. **Health and Wellness**
   - **Example**: *Lose 10 pounds in three months by doing 30 minutes of exercise five days a week and tracking food intake.*
   - **Possible Action Steps**: *Join a gym or a dance class, meal-prep on Sundays, reduce sugary drinks.*
2. **Professional Growth**
   - **Example**: *Earn a specific certification within six months to become eligible for a promotion.*
   - **Action Steps**: *Enroll in an online course, allocate two study hours daily, practice mock exams monthly.*
3. **Communication Skills**
   - **Example**: *Become more assertive in work meetings over three months, speaking up at least once in every team discussion.*
   - **Action Steps**: *Prepare talking points before meetings, ask a colleague for feedback, practice with a friend.*
4. **Creative Pursuits**
   - **Example**: *Write a short story collection in one year, finishing one story per month.*
   - **Action Steps**: *Set aside three writing sessions weekly, attend a local writers' group, read a craft book every quarter.*

5. **Financial Stability**
    - **Example**: Build an emergency fund covering three months of expenses within eight months.
    - **Action Steps**: Create a budget, cut unnecessary subscriptions, track spending weekly, automatically transfer a set amount to savings.

Each example can be further customized with timelines, milestones, and specific measurement tools. The essence is translating your aspirations into a structured framework.

19.12 Handling Fear and Doubt in the Development Process

Even with a clear plan, fear or doubt might creep in:

1. **Normalize Fear**
    - **Reason**: Growth often involves stepping outside comfort zones. Fear indicates you are challenging yourself.
    - **Perspective**: Remind yourself that small anxieties can be harnessed as energy to be more prepared and careful.
2. **Mindset Shifts**
    - **From Failure to Learning**: If something does not go as planned, reflect on what you can learn instead of labeling it a defeat.
    - **From Perfection to Progress**: Aim for consistent improvement rather than flawlessness.
3. **Support System**
    - **Encouragement**: Share concerns with a friend, mentor, or group who can validate your feelings and offer solutions.
    - **Role Models**: Look up to people who overcame similar fears. They prove it is possible to triumph over self-doubt.
4. **Practical Stress Management**
    - **Relaxation Techniques**: Breathing exercises, short meditations, or gentle stretches can calm nerves when you feel overwhelmed.
    - **Incremental Exposure**: If you fear public speaking, start with smaller audiences or mini-presentations to reduce anxiety gradually.

Facing fear with an open mind builds resilience, another cornerstone of confidence.

19.13 Using Visualization and Affirmations

Tools like visualization and affirmations can reinforce your determination:

1. **Visualization**
   - **Technique**: *Close your eyes and picture yourself accomplishing a specific step—like delivering an impressive presentation or crossing a marathon finish line. Notice the details: how you look, feel, and act.*
   - **Benefit**: *Rehearsing success in your mind primes you to feel more comfortable and confident in real-life scenarios.*
2. **Affirmations**
   - **Short, Positive Statements**: *For instance, "I am fully capable of learning new skills" or "I handle challenges with resilience."*
   - **Repetition**: *Repeat them daily—on waking, during breaks, or before bed—so they gradually replace negative inner chatter.*
3. **Belief System**
   - **Self-Fulfilling**: *When you believe you can succeed, you are more likely to notice opportunities and persist through obstacles.*
   - **Personalize**: *Choose wording that resonates with you personally. Affirmations should feel authentic, not empty slogans.*

Though they may seem simple, visualization and affirmations can significantly strengthen your resolve to follow through with the steps in your personal development plan.

19.14 Accountability and External Feedback

Staying accountable keeps you honest about progress and can offer fresh perspectives:

1. **Accountability Partners**
    - **Mutual Check-Ins**: Agree to meet or message weekly, reviewing each other's goals, achievements, and challenges.
    - **Support and Challenge**: Offer encouragement but also question excuses if they see patterns of procrastination.
2. **Mentors or Coaches**
    - **Expert Guidance**: If you can afford it, a coach offers tailored strategies for your plan. Mentors with experience in your goal area can also provide targeted advice.
    - **Progress Reviews**: Schedule monthly calls to discuss achievements, setbacks, or any needed course corrections.
3. **Peer Groups**
    - **Online or Offline**: Join groups where members share similar goals—like fitness communities, writing circles, or professional associations.
    - **Collective Energy**: Group enthusiasm can motivate you when personal willpower is low.
4. **Sharing Milestones Publicly**
    - **Pros and Cons**: Announcing goals on social media can spur you to follow through. But be mindful—public scrutiny can add pressure.
    - **Choose Wisely**: If social platforms might cause undue stress, consider a smaller, more supportive circle instead.

Healthy accountability fosters a sense that you are not alone, motivating you to stay on track and learn from external observations.

19.15 Celebrating Growth: Internal Shifts as Well as External Achievements

Personal development includes both visible milestones (like finishing a certificate program) and inner growth (like feeling calmer in stressful situations). Recognize intangible wins:

1. **Transformation Markers**
    - **Examples**: "I handle criticism more calmly now," or "I'm no longer intimidated by networking events."

- **Journaling**: Writing down these internal shifts highlights how much your mindset or emotional state has evolved.
2. **Confidence Indicators**
    - **Self-Expression**: You speak up more in group discussions or share your ideas confidently online.
    - **Better Boundaries**: You can say "no" to unreasonable demands without guilt.
3. **Attitude Changes**
    - **Optimistic Outlook**: You feel more hopeful about solving problems.
    - **Self-Compassion**: You judge yourself less harshly for mistakes, focusing on learning instead.
4. **Improved Relationships**
    - **Communication**: Notice if conflicts resolve more smoothly or you show deeper empathy to loved ones.
    - **Quality Interactions**: You connect with people more genuinely because you feel at ease in your own skin.

Tracking these internal transformations is essential because they often form the very essence of self-confidence. While external achievements can be measured, these subtle personal victories also deserve acknowledgment.

19.16 Integrating Your Plan with Everyday Life

Your personal development plan works best when it fits naturally into your daily routines:

1. **Embed Tasks into Existing Habits**
    - **"Habit Stacking"**: If you already have a habit of enjoying morning tea, use that time to read a few pages relevant to your goal or do a quick journaling exercise.
    - **Align with Schedules**: If you are an early riser, place creative or demanding tasks in the morning. If you are a night owl, maybe schedule learning time after dinner.
2. **Use Micro-Moments**
    - **Commutes**: Listen to audiobooks or podcasts that support your goals.

- **Waiting Periods**: While waiting at the doctor's office, draft an outline of your next step or research an upcoming milestone.
3. **Family or Roommate Involvement**
    - **Mutual Support**: If others in your household also have goals, plan times to work quietly side by side or share tips.
    - **Friendly Reminders**: Loved ones can gently nudge you if they notice you slipping from your plan.
4. **Gently Self-Check**
    - **Daily Review**: Before bed, ask, "Did I make progress on my plan today? If not, why?"
    - **Adjust Tomorrow**: Based on your reflection, make small changes for the next day's approach.

When your plan seamlessly blends with your lifestyle, it becomes a natural aspect of your day instead of an extra burden.

19.17 Revising or Renewing Your Personal Development Plan

Over time, you will accomplish some goals, lose interest in others, or discover brand-new directions. Periodically refine your plan:

1. **Regular Audits**
    - **Every 3–6 Months**: Review your entire personal development plan. Which goals are still relevant? Have your values or life circumstances shifted?
    - **Achievements**: Tick off what you have completed, and note any lessons learned.
2. **Add or Replace Goals**
    - **Completion**: Once you have hit a major goal, you might add a new one.
    - **Discard**: If a goal no longer resonates, remove it rather than dragging it along and feeling guilty.
3. **Reset Timelines**
    - **Speed Up**: If you are moving faster than expected, you can accelerate certain deadlines.
    - **Slow Down**: If you are behind, push the timeline out a bit—this is not failure, but practical realism.
4. **Celebrate or Transition**

- ○ **Milestone Moments**: With each plan refresh, celebrate your achievements.
- ○ **New Phases**: Goals you have outgrown might lead you to more advanced or different challenges. Accept this evolution as a positive sign of growth.

Refreshes keep your personal development plan dynamic, mirroring your current stage in life and ensuring you stay passionate and aligned with your ever-evolving self.

19.18 Example of a Simple Personal Development Plan Outline

Here is a hypothetical outline to illustrate how you might arrange your own plan:

- **Date Started**: January 1, 20XX
- **Time Frame**: 6 months (with monthly reviews)
1. **Goal #1**: Improve Public Speaking
    - ○ **Why**: To feel more confident in work presentations and social events.
    - ○ **Actions**:
        - Join Toastmasters or a local speaking club.
        - Practice a 3-minute talk at home weekly.
        - Volunteer to present one short report at work by March.
    - ○ **Milestones**:
        - 1st talk at Toastmasters by February 1.
        - Work presentation by March 15.
    - ○ **Measure**:
        - Comfort level rated 1–10 before and after each speech.
        - Feedback from colleagues.
2. **Goal #2**: Start a Healthy Eating Routine
    - ○ **Why**: Boost energy, improve long-term wellness.
    - ○ **Actions**:
        - Plan weekly meal menus every Sunday.
        - Swap sugary snacks for fruit or yogurt.
        - Track water intake daily (aim for 8 cups).

- **Milestones**:
    - Maintain the habit for 4 consecutive weeks.
    - Visit a nutritionist by April for advice.
- **Measure**:
    - Weight check once a month, energy levels self-rated weekly.

3. **Goal #3**: Deepen Creative Skills (Painting)
   - **Why**: Increase personal fulfillment and relax from work stress.
   - **Actions**:
     - Enroll in a beginner's painting course by February.
     - Dedicate 2 hours each weekend to painting.
     - Share finished pieces with a supportive friend or online group for feedback.
   - **Milestones**:
     - Complete first painting by March 1.
     - Participate in a small local art display or online showcase by July.
   - **Measure**:
     - Number of paintings completed, skill improvement noticed by self or friends.

4. **Review Schedule**:
   - **Monthly Check**: Last Saturday of each month to assess progress, note challenges, and adjust tasks.

5. **End-of-Plan Assessment (July)**:
   - Evaluate achievements, celebrate successes, decide next steps or new goals.

This example shows how you might structure your plan with clarity and accountability. The details—timelines, tasks, measures—keep you on track, while the reflection points give you space to adapt.

19.19 Motivational Mindset: Rewarding Yourself Along the Way

Consistency can be challenging if the journey feels like a long marathon with no breaks. Rewarding yourself at strategic intervals keeps morale high:

1. **Tangible Treats**

- **Small Indulgences**: A new book, a fancy tea, or a treat from a local bakery after completing a milestone.
- **Bigger Celebrations**: An overnight trip, a spa appointment, or buying a cherished item after finishing a major goal.

2. **Experiential Rewards**
   - **Leisure Activities**: A day hike, painting in a scenic park, or attending a music event.
   - **Gathering with Friends**: Have a simple get-together to share your latest success, letting them enjoy your excitement with you.
3. **Tracking and Visual Cues**
   - **Progress Chart**: Mark a star or sticker each time you complete a micro-goal.
   - **Symbols of Achievement**: Keep a jar where you drop a marble for every step you accomplish. Watch it fill up over time.
4. **Emotional Rewards**
   - **Affirming Statements**: Congratulate yourself out loud or in a journal: "I made it this far—I can keep going!"
   - **Self-Gratitude**: Thank yourself for the effort, reinforcing self-love and worthiness.

Even small rewards can transform a tough or tedious task into a satisfying challenge. This positive reinforcement system helps you stay enthusiastic from one milestone to the next.

CHAPTER 20

Celebrating Progress and Planning for the Future

20.1 Introduction: The Journey Continues

Completing this book does not mark the end of your confidence-building journey. Rather, it is another stepping stone on the path of continuous growth. You have absorbed insights on understanding confidence, handling obstacles, nurturing self-care, building relationships, mentoring others, and now creating a personal development plan. The logical next step is to celebrate how far you have come and consider where you would like to go next.

This chapter focuses on the dual objectives of commemorating your accomplishments—both large and small—and planning future moves that sustain your newfound confidence. Life is not static; as you achieve goals, new ambitions emerge. As you surmount challenges, fresh ones appear. By learning to pause and celebrate each stage, then lay a strategic blueprint for what is ahead, you maintain momentum and keep expanding your comfort zone. It is a cycle of growth: reflect, celebrate, adapt, plan, and move forward.

20.2 Why Celebration Matters

Many women push themselves relentlessly, achieving goal after goal, yet never stop to acknowledge their own success. Over time, this can lead to burnout or a sense of emptiness. Proper celebration is vital for multiple reasons:

1. **Emotional Reward**
   - **Positive Reinforcement**: Acknowledging a win—like completing a tough course or resolving a long-standing conflict—releases feel-good emotions, reinforcing your confidence.
   - **Motivation**: Celebrations act as mental checkpoints that inspire you to tackle bigger or new targets.
2. **Stress Relief**

- **Pause and Relax**: Celebrations allow you to exhale, enjoy the moment, and decompress from the hard work you invested.
- **Improved Well-Being**: Recognizing success fosters gratitude and can reduce the anxiety of "What's next?"

3. **Sense of Progress**
   - **Self-Affirmation**: You realize you are not stuck; you are evolving. This self-awareness combats doubts about "Have I really changed?"
   - **Clarity**: Assessing what you did to succeed helps you refine techniques for future goals.
4. **Community Building**
   - **Shared Joy**: Inviting friends or family to celebrate fosters deeper bonds. They see your progress and share in your happiness.
   - **Inspiration**: Your success story might encourage someone else to pursue their own dreams.

Celebration does not have to be extravagant or costly. Even small gestures—like a toast with loved ones or a relaxing afternoon dedicated to a cherished hobby—can mark the significance of your growth.

20.3 Acknowledging Internal Transformations

It is easy to focus on external achievements like promotions, weight loss goals, or completing a creative project. But internal shifts are equally important:

1. **Emotional Milestones**
   - **Reduced Negative Self-Talk**: If you catch yourself criticizing less or using kinder language towards yourself, that is progress.
   - **Calmer Reactions**: Moments when you handle stress or confrontation with newfound composure indicate deeper emotional resilience.
2. **Improved Boundaries and Self-Advocacy**
   - **Speaking Up**: Maybe you requested better work conditions or said "no" to an unreasonable favor. That is a big internal win.

- **Balanced Relationships**: *If a previously strained relationship is healthier because you stood up for your needs, celebrate that step.*
3. **Mindset Shifts**
    - **Growth Mindset**: *Adopting the belief that abilities and intelligence can be developed. For example, you tried an unfamiliar skill and realized mistakes are part of learning.*
    - **Optimism**: *Maybe you consciously replaced "I can't" with "I can learn how."*
4. **Confidence Indicators**
    - **Openness to Challenges**: *Observing that you take risks more readily than before—like volunteering to lead a new project or sign up for a public speaking event.*
    - **Respecting Self-Care**: *Recognizing that rest and self-nurturing are essential, not indulgent.*

Create moments to reflect on these intangible wins, because they serve as the backbone of long-term self-confidence.

20.4 Methods of Celebration That Suit Different Lifestyles

Celebrations come in all shapes and sizes. You can tailor them to your personality, available time, and resources:

1. **Solitary Reflection**
    - **Quiet Gratitude**: *Spend an hour alone in a peaceful setting—like a park or a cozy room—thinking about your progress.*
    - **Journaling**: *Write a "celebration entry," describing recent triumphs, large or small, and how they make you feel.*
2. **Group Activities**
    - **Friends' Gathering**: *Invite a few close friends for a simple dinner, acknowledging the goal or milestone. Let them know what they are celebrating with you.*
    - **Family Outing**: *Plan a fun weekend trip or a local adventure. Emphasize that it is to mark your personal milestone.*
3. **Symbolic Gestures**

- **Certificate or Keepsake**: Design or purchase a small token (like a bracelet or a charm) representing your achievement. Each time you see it, you remember your growth.
- **Planting**: Some people plant a tree or flowers, symbolizing new beginnings and continued growth.

4. **Pampering and Relaxation**
   - **Spa Day or Massage**: Physical relaxation can help you slow down and appreciate how far you have come.
   - **Hobby Indulgence**: If you love reading, buy a new novel and spend a day leisurely exploring it without guilt.

The point is not extravagance but the mindful act of pausing to say, "I did something meaningful, and I deserve to honor it."

20.5 Sharing Your Progress with Supportive Circles

Your achievements might inspire others or lead to valuable feedback:

1. **Trusted Friends or Mentors**
   - **Small Circle**: A casual update—like a group message or a conversation—lets them celebrate with you and offer congratulations.
   - **Mentor Feedback**: A mentor's perspective on your growth can provide fresh insights and encouragement for next steps.
2. **Social Media**
   - **Platform Choice**: Some prefer more professional platforms (like LinkedIn) for career successes, while others share personal achievements on Facebook or Instagram.
   - **Modesty vs. Pride**: If you worry about appearing boastful, focus on the process and lessons learned. People often appreciate authenticity.
3. **Community or Online Groups**
   - **Forums and Workshops**: If you belong to a group that discusses self-improvement, let them know your recent milestones. You might spark a motivating discussion.
   - **Reciprocal Support**: Hearing others' success stories and returning the praise fosters a culture of mutual uplift.

Balancing humility with recognition of your hard work can open doors to new opportunities and deeper connections. Do not be afraid to let people see how you have grown—most will cheer you on.

20.6 Transitioning from Achieved Goals to New Ambitions

After hitting a major milestone—like completing a personal development plan or mastering a skill—it is tempting to relax indefinitely. While rest is vital, you can harness your current momentum to build new, fulfilling challenges:

1. **Reflect on Lessons**
    - **What Worked**: Which strategies or routines propelled you to success? You might replicate them for your next goal.
    - **What Changed**: Have your interests shifted? Did you realize you prefer learning in a group setting or alone? Let these realizations guide future plans.
2. **Next-Level Aspirations**
    - **Building On Wins**: If you finished a beginner language course, perhaps you aim for conversational fluency next. If you ran a 5K, maybe you aim for a 10K.
    - **Branching Out**: Sometimes a completed goal reveals a new path—like turning a writing hobby into a side business.
3. **Fresh Timelines**
    - **Realistic Start**: Do not rush. Give yourself time to re-energize before diving into a new challenge.
    - **Overlap**: If your new goal naturally complements existing roles (like family or work), plan how to integrate it smoothly.
4. **Evolving Identity**
    - **Confidence Cascade**: Achieving one goal often makes you realize you are capable of more than you once believed. This renewed self-esteem can fuel bolder ambitions.
    - **Guard Against Complacency**: While celebrating, remain open to the idea that you can continue growing in different directions. Life is full of surprises.

Leverage your recent accomplishment as a launching pad. The sense of capability you gained can help you tackle fresh dreams with optimism.

20.7 Sustaining Confidence in Changing Environments

Life circumstances often shift—jobs evolve, relationships change, health needs fluctuate. Your confidence can waver if you tie it solely to stable conditions. Instead:

1. **Adapt Your Strategies**
    - **Flexible Goals**: If you unexpectedly move to a new city, adapt your career or relationship goals to that location's realities.
    - **Skill Transfer**: Embrace a mindset that your core skills—communication, problem-solving, leadership—remain valuable in any environment.
2. **Use Setbacks as Launchpads**
    - **Learning Mindset**: A lost opportunity might prompt you to explore new paths. A job layoff could lead to pursuing that dream business.
    - **Emotional Resilience**: Remind yourself of past triumphs over adversity. If you overcame obstacles before, you can do it again.
3. **Maintain Core Practices**
    - **Routine Anchors**: Keep certain confidence-boosting habits—like journaling or short workouts—consistent, even during upheaval.
    - **Support Network**: Lean on friends, mentors, or professional advice to navigate big changes more calmly.
4. **Celebrate Small Victories in Transitions**
    - **Micro-Accomplishments**: If you move to a new country, simply learning a few local phrases or setting up your living space can be mini goals worth celebrating.
    - **Reinforce Self-Concept**: Each step forward cements your identity as someone who can adapt and thrive.

Sustaining confidence means trusting your ability to adjust. Growth does not stop because life gets complicated—it merely changes shape.

20.8 The Ongoing Role of Self-Care and Well-Being

Confidence is intertwined with wellness. As you keep pursuing dreams, do not neglect rest and emotional health:

1. **Physical Health**
   - **Activity Balance**: Maintain some form of regular exercise or movement that you enjoy. A strong body supports a strong mind.
   - **Nutrition and Sleep**: Balanced meals and sufficient rest keep your energy high and mood stable.
2. **Mental Health Checks**
   - **Stress Management**: If you sense burnout, scale back, delegate tasks, or try mindfulness techniques to decompress.
   - **Professional Help**: Therapists or counselors can guide you through tough emotional periods, preventing deeper crises.
3. **Boundaries in Relationships**
   - **Protect Energy**: Surround yourself with people who respect your time and growth rather than those who drain you.
   - **Communication**: Politely but firmly handle requests that exceed your capacity. Explain your need to preserve personal space.
4. **Fun and Leisure**
   - **Hobbies**: Keep at least one purely enjoyable pastime—reading fiction, gardening, crafting—unrelated to productivity or goals.
   - **Mini Escapes**: Plan occasional day trips or weekend getaways to refresh your perspective.

When self-care becomes part of your identity, you equip yourself with the resilience required for ongoing confidence and achievement.

20.9 Mentoring Others as a Means of Growth

Having invested effort into building your own confidence, you can reinforce it further by helping others—a concept explored in Chapter 18. But let us revisit how it ties specifically to future planning:

1. **Sharing Knowledge**

- **Teaching**: Explaining how you overcame self-doubt or mastered certain skills benefits both you and your listeners. Teaching cements your own learning.
- **Encouraging**: By cheering someone else on, you remind yourself of the steps you took and your capacity to succeed again.

2. **Mutual Learning**
    - **Fresh Insights**: A mentee's questions can challenge you to clarify your thinking, sometimes leading to new personal goals.
    - **Network Expansion**: Mentoring fosters a support network that may open unexpected doors for your future endeavors.

3. **Legacy and Community**
    - **Positive Impact**: Knowing you made a difference in someone's life can be a powerful motivator to keep striving for excellence.
    - **Role Modeling**: Your own growth story can spark a ripple effect, inspiring other women to chase their dreams.

Serving as a mentor or guide is not only a generous act but also a strategic move to maintain and deepen your confidence by revisiting the lessons you have learned.

20.10 Crafting a Vision for the Future

As you progress, you might find it helpful to form a longer-term vision of what you want your life to look like in 5, 10, or 20 years:

1. **Imaginative Exercise**
    - **Dream Freely**: Let go of practicality for a moment. Picture your ideal day, environment, relationships, and achievements.
    - **Sensory Detail**: Notice what you see, hear, and feel. This vividness can boost motivation.
2. **Align with Values**
    - **Cross-Check**: Does your future vision resonate with your core values—like community, family, adventure, or creativity? If not, refine it.
    - **Emotional Indicators**: If certain goals feel dull, they might not belong in your vision, or you need to link them to something personally meaningful.

3. **Reverse Engineering**
    - **Break It Down**: From the 10-year vision, step backward. What must you achieve in the next 5 years, 2 years, or 6 months to move in that direction?
    - **Realism and Flexibility**: The plan is not set in stone; it simply offers a sense of direction so your daily actions build toward your ultimate dreams.
4. **Reflecting on Current Path**
    - **Adjusting**: If your present career or habits do not align with the future you imagine, consider how to pivot gradually—maybe through additional education, new job prospects, or different relationship patterns.

A forward-looking vision keeps your confidence alive by reminding you that each day's actions contribute to a broader, self-defined destiny.

20.11 Involving Loved Ones in Future Plans

Confidence flourishes when the people around you support your endeavors. Consider how to include them:

1. **Shared Goals**
    - **Collaborative Projects**: If you and your partner both want better health, create a joint fitness plan. If you and a friend aim to learn painting, enroll in classes together.
    - **Family Vision**: If you have kids, discuss family dreams—like traveling or moving to a bigger home—so everyone feels invested.
2. **Seeking Their Input**
    - **Open Conversations**: Talk about your aspirations with loved ones, inviting their thoughts or suggestions.
    - **Constructive Criticism**: If they see potential blind spots, listening might refine your plan.
3. **Respecting Boundaries**
    - **Personal vs. Collective**: Some goals—like spiritual growth or career shifts—are personal. Seek support but remain true to your own convictions.

- **Encouragement Not Control**: Loved ones may have opinions on your direction; weigh them, but keep final decisions aligned with your self-knowledge.

When your circle understands and endorses your vision, their cheerleading and practical help can bolster your confidence significantly.

20.12 Reflecting on Lessons Learned from This Journey

Throughout this book, you have encountered diverse topics—inner critic management, self-care, boundary setting, assertiveness, emotional resilience, positive thinking, communication skills, stress management, self-awareness, goal-setting, relationships, self-care, etc. Summarizing key takeaways ensures you do not lose the lessons:

1. **Confidence Is Multifaceted**
   - **Ongoing Process**: It is not a one-time achievement but a skill you cultivate repeatedly in various life areas.
2. **Mindset and Action**
   - **Intertwined**: Positive thinking, visualization, and self-affirmations help shift your mindset, but concrete action—like stepping out of your comfort zone—reinforces those mental changes.
3. **Balance and Self-Care**
   - **Prevent Overwhelm**: Overloading yourself or ignoring personal well-being can erode confidence and hamper long-term growth.
4. **Support Networks**
   - **Collaborative**: Friends, mentors, colleagues, and family can catalyze or hinder your progress, so choose relationships wisely.
5. **Learning from Obstacles**
   - **Resilience**: Facing challenges is inevitable. The real growth lies in how you handle and learn from them.

As you plan future goals and direction, keep these principles at the forefront. They act as cornerstones for every new phase of personal evolution.

20.13 Sustaining the Lessons Beyond This Book

Finishing this book may bring a sense of completion, but real transformation depends on how you apply its principles daily:

1. **Revisit Chapters as Needed**
    - **Topical Review**: If you encounter a specific issue—like setting boundaries or dealing with stress—re-skim the relevant chapter to refresh strategies.
    - **Consistency**: Sometimes life derails good habits. Briefly returning to certain passages can realign your mindset.
2. **Practice Over Theory**
    - **Daily Implementation**: Integrate small habits from the book—like using "I" statements, managing fear, or practicing gratitude—into your routines.
    - **Challenge Yourself**: Each week, pick one tip or technique from a chapter to apply in real situations.
3. **Continue Expanding Knowledge**
    - **Further Reading**: Explore other books or resources recommended within or outside the topics covered here—like specialized works on leadership, emotional intelligence, or financial health.
    - **Workshops and Courses**: Reinforce your progress with structured learning experiences to deepen certain skill sets.

The more consistently you practice, the more natural these confidence-building methods become, eventually shaping your default way of being.

20.14 Long-Term Vision: Becoming a Lifelong Learner

Confidence thrives in those who see themselves as perpetual students of life:

1. **Embrace Curiosity**

- **Questions**: Keep asking "Why?" or "How?" in everyday life—like exploring why certain habits stick or how you can improve your environment.
- **Try New Things**: Accept invitations to experiences outside your usual comfort zone, fueling growth.

2. **Adapt and Renew**
    - **Technological and Social Changes**: The world evolves quickly, so adopt a mindset of flexibility. Enjoy learning new software, discovering cultural trends, or shifting career paths.
    - **Upgrading Beliefs**: If you find old convictions no longer serve you, replace them with updated perspectives that match your current reality and knowledge.
3. **Mentor the Next Wave**
    - **Pay It Forward**: As you deepen your learning, sharing with others cements your knowledge and fosters a culture of collective growth.
    - **Continual Improvement**: Teaching or guiding ensures you remain engaged and up-to-date.

Sustained confidence arises from recognizing that learning never ends. Each stage in life unveils fresh challenges and joys, fueling ongoing empowerment.

20.15 Dealing with Future Setbacks

No matter how well you plan, future setbacks will appear—be it health issues, job loss, relationship strains, or global events. Prepare for them:

1. **Resilience Toolkit**
    - **Coping Strategies**: Keep practicing mindfulness, journaling, or seeking professional help if stress levels soar.
    - **Financial Preparedness**: Building an emergency fund or having multiple career skills can buffer unexpected changes.
2. **Perspective Shifts**
    - **Temporary**: Remind yourself that difficulties, while painful, are often temporary phases.
    - **Learning Lens**: Ask, "What can this setback teach me about my strengths or weaknesses?"
3. **Pivot Gracefully**

- **Adapt Plans**: If a major life event hinders certain goals, re-evaluate timelines or tweak objectives.
- **Focus on Well-Being**: Sometimes you must suspend ambitious projects to handle crises. That is okay; you can restart later.

Each setback is an invitation to reinforce your confidence by adapting, learning, and eventually bouncing back stronger than before.

20.16 Fostering Hope for Ongoing Transformation

Confidence also involves hope—the belief in better outcomes ahead:

1. **Hope vs. Unrealistic Expectations**
    - **Balanced Optimism**: You accept that achieving goals may be difficult but remain confident in your perseverance and resourcefulness.
    - **Action-Oriented**: True hope spurs you to act, not just wish.
2. **Visualizing a Brighter Future**
    - **Mental Pictures**: Similar to Chapter 19's discussion on visualization, imagine yourself thriving years from now.
    - **Hope as Fuel**: When motivation dips, recall that hopeful image to reignite your commitment.
3. **Stories of Triumph**
    - **Look to Role Models**: People who overcame adversity provide living evidence that hope can manifest into reality through determination.
    - **Your Own Wins**: Reflect on past victories—however small—to reaffirm your ability to achieve more.

Hopeful thinking fosters resilience and keeps you forging ahead through uncertain times, trusting in your capacity for transformation.

20.17 Cultivating Gratitude Alongside Confidence

Gratitude and confidence work together beautifully. While confidence pushes you to believe in your capabilities, gratitude reminds you of the support, resources, and opportunities that made your journey possible:

1. **Daily Gratitude Practices**
    - **Quick Lists**: Each morning or evening, jot down 3–5 things you are thankful for—like a sunny day, a kind coworker, or the chance to learn something new.
    - **Deeper Reflection**: Occasionally pick one item and explore why it matters so much in your life.
2. **Acknowledging Helpers**
    - **Express Appreciation**: Thank mentors, friends, or family members who contributed to your success.
    - **Pay It Forward**: If someone assisted your growth, consider doing something thoughtful for them or for others in similar situations.
3. **Grateful for Challenges**
    - **Reframing**: Even obstacles can be blessings in disguise—helping you develop patience, creativity, or empathy.
    - **Learning Mindset**: Gratitude for lessons learned fosters a calm acceptance of life's ups and downs.

Feeling grateful cements your sense of abundance. You realize that while you are strong on your own, you thrive even more with the blessings of supportive people, environments, or moments.

20.18 Sustaining Momentum: Routines and Systems

Confidence can wane if you do not integrate your new approaches into daily life. Systems and routines keep your progress steady:

1. **Morning Rituals**
    - **Positive Start**: Begin each day with a small act—like reading an affirmation, doing gentle stretches, or reviewing your day's top goals.

- **Mental Clarity**: This sets a proactive tone, reminding you of your purpose and reinforcing confidence.
2. **Evening Wind-Down**
    - **Reflection Time**: Before bed, note any achievements or insights. If you encountered setbacks, outline a quick plan for tomorrow.
    - **Relaxation**: Wind down with calming activities, ensuring better sleep and mental refreshment.
3. **Weekly or Monthly Planning**
    - **Batch Tasks**: Group similar tasks (like paying bills or scheduling appointments) on specific days to reduce mental clutter.
    - **Consistent Reviews**: Check your personal development plan to see if you are on track or need adjustments.
4. **Accountability Checkpoints**
    - **Regular Meetings**: If you have an accountability partner or group, keep those sessions in your calendar.
    - **Visual Boards**: Update your vision board or progress chart weekly, watching your momentum grow.

Routines make confidence-building almost automatic. With each repeated habit, you reinforce a stable, self-assured identity.

20.19 Gratitude for Yourself and Forward Focus

At this point, you have journeyed through insights, strategies, exercises, and reflective processes to nurture a strong, enduring confidence. It is time to acknowledge yourself for the dedication and bravery it took to confront old doubts, adopt healthier habits, and try new ideas:

1. **Commend Your Effort**
    - **Self-Praise**: You are allowed to say, "I am proud of the work I have done and who I am becoming."
    - **Highlight Specific Steps**: Cite particular changes—like learning to set boundaries or starting a personal development plan.
2. **Recognize Imperfections**
    - **Acceptance**: There will still be days of insecurity or stress. That does not negate your progress.

- **Continuation**: Confidence is not about never feeling doubt; it is about forging ahead despite it.
3. **Look Ahead**
    - **Recommitment**: Affirm your commitment to keep learning, refining your personal development plan, and helping others if possible.
    - **Positive Anticipation**: Imagine the new opportunities, relationships, and breakthroughs that may arise as you keep nurturing your confidence.

As you appreciate how far you have come, you pave the way for further achievements and deeper self-trust.

20.20 Conclusion

Celebrating your progress and planning for the future encapsulates the essence of ongoing confidence and personal growth. By consciously marking your milestones—both internal and external—you feed your motivation and sense of accomplishment. Simultaneously, looking forward with a practical plan ensures that your newfound self-belief does not remain stagnant. Instead, it evolves alongside your changing life circumstances.

This final chapter affirms that your journey does not stop here. Armed with the strategies from this book, you can continue adjusting your self-care routines, communication skills, goal-setting methods, mentoring capabilities, and overall mindset. As you do, remember to pause regularly—applaud your efforts, reflect on lessons, and connect the dots between past wins and future endeavors. Such a cycle of celebrating what is and anticipating what can be sustains a powerful sense of confidence that grows richer with each new phase of life.

As you close this book, you stand at a fresh beginning rather than an endpoint. Embrace the excitement of continued learning, remain kind to yourself when facing detours, and trust that your capacity to grow is boundless. May each victory—tiny or grand—strengthen your conviction that you are capable of transformation, worthy of your goals, and prepared to inspire others along the way. Your personal growth story is ongoing, and every page you write next is infused with the optimism, resilience, and confident spirit you have cultivated here.

www.ingramcontent.com/pod-product-compliance
Lightning Source LLC
LaVergne TN
LVHW012038070526
838202LV00056B/5532